Living Well with Heart Disease

Living Well with
HEART DISEASE

Cardiovascular Services, Fairview Health Services,
affiliated with the University of Minnesota

Fairview Press • Minneapolis

Published by Fairview Press, 2450 Riverside Avenue, Minneapolis, Minnesota 55454.

Library of Congress Cataloging-in-Publication Data
Living well with heart disease / Cardiovascular Services [Unit], Fairview Health Services, affiliated with the University of Minnesota.
    p. cm.
  Includes bibliographical references and index.
  ISBN 1-57749-089-4 (pb : alk. paper)
   1. Heart—Diseases—Popular works. I. Fairview Health Services. Cardiovascular Services Unit.

  RC672.L56 2000
  616.1'2—dc21   99-047418

First Printing: January 2000

Printed in the United States of America
03 02 01 00   5 4 3 2 1

Writer: Linda Picone
Cover: *Cover Design by Laurie Ingram Duren*™
Interior design: Jane Dahms Nicolo
Illustrations: Barbara Beshoar and Jane Dahms Nicolo

For a free catalog of Fairview Press titles, please call toll-free 1-800-544-8207. Or visit our web site at *www.Press.Fairview.org*.

This book is dedicated to patients and families who experience cardiac disease, and to the cardiac care providers who make a difference in their lives.

ACKNOWLEDGMENTS

Fairview is a community-focused health system providing a complete range of services, from prevention of illness and injury to care for the most complex medical conditions. The information contained in this book was assembled and developed by our cardiovascular team.

Many individuals from Fairview Health Services contributed to this project. They include Wayne Aakre, RDCS; Carol Bauer; Nancy Breazile, CT; Jennifer Breeding, PharmD; Duane Brook, RDCS; Richard Clark, BA, CVT/EP; Shirley Hagen, RN; Janet Heisterman, RN, MN; William Hession, MD; Carolyn Howland, BS, CNMT; Terri Kinowski, RN, BSN, CCRN; Janelle Lawler, RD, LD; Kristen McWilliams, OTR/CES; Pat Nord, RN, BSN, CCRN; Michael Petty, RN, MS, CCRN; Julie Sabo, RN, MN, CCRN; Laura Schuerman, RN, BSN; Elaine Stevens, RN, MSN, CCRN; Janell Strohshane, PharmD; Barbara Van Hauer, RN, BSN; Melissa Van Holland, PharmD; Paula Varhol, RN, BS; and Dorinda Vloo, RN, BSN.

CONTENTS

INTRODUCTION

If you've picked up this book, chances are you—or someone close to you—has already had a heart problem. Maybe it's an occasional irregular heartbeat. Maybe it's a sense of fatigue and shortness of breath. Maybe a full-blown heart attack.

Any sign of heart trouble can be frightening. Indeed, some heart problems are life threatening. But thanks to modern medicine and a greater understanding of how lifestyle choices can affect the heart, your chances of living a long and happy life with a heart problem are far better than they were ten years ago.

To get the best treatment for your heart, the expertise and recommendations of your healthcare providers are crucial. But something else is crucial as well:

Your involvement in your own healthcare.

This means:

- Understanding your diagnosis.

- Asking questions if you don't understand something.

- Getting more information about your heart problem.

- Exploring the full range of options for your treatment.

Being involved in your own healthcare also means following through with treatment and lifestyle changes. You must be active in building and maintaining a healthier heart for the rest of your life. You may have to take medication every day, change your diet, stop smoking, lose weight, reduce stress, and exercise regularly. Although medical advances have been considerable in recent years, for most people, personal effort is the key to preventing, overcoming, and recovering from heart disease.

This book is intended for people who are under a doctor's care for heart problems. It is designed to help you understand the basics about how the heart functions, heart disease, treatment options, and the steps to recovery.

Since the book covers a broad range of heart diseases and treatments, some parts of this book may not apply to you. Use the book as a reference, reading chapters—or parts of chapters—that affect you or your family.

CHAPTER ONE

UNDERSTANDING YOUR HEART

Most people are more familiar with the heart than with any other organ in the body; yet, they are sometimes off-base about what the heart does and how it functions.

In this chapter you will learn:

How your heart works.

The role of the circulatory system.

Where the coronary arteries are located and what they do.

What we mean by the term "blood pressure."

How the heart valves work.

THE HEART IS A MUSCLE

How does the
heart work?

The heart is a muscle that works like a pump. It's about the size of your fist and shaped something like a pear, rather than like the traditional "heart shape" we see on Valentine's Day cards. As your heart pumps, it takes nutrients and oxygen to all parts of your body, while picking up waste products produced by your cells. The heart lies predominately on the left side of the breastbone.

In one day, your heart will beat about 100,000 times, moving the equivalent of about 2,000 gallons of blood.

Your heart is actually a double pump with four chambers. On top are the right atrium and the left atrium; on the bottom are the right ventricle and the left ventricle.

Blood comes into the heart through the right atrium, then flows into the right ventricle. The right ventricle pumps the blood through the pulmonary artery to the lungs, where it absorbs fresh oxygen. The blood, now full of oxygen, goes back to the heart, where it collects in the left atrium. It then flows into the left ventricle and is pumped into the aorta, which carries the blood to the rest of the body.

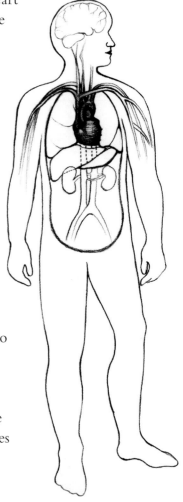

The heart's position in the body.

When your heart beats, both atria (plural of atrium) contract, forcing blood into the ventricles. The valves between the atria and the ventricles close. Then the ventricles contract, forcing blood through another set of valves into the lungs and the rest of the body. This second set of valves closes. Therefore, in one heartbeat, blood moves through two parts of the heart, with valves closing behind each movement.

Atria Filling
Blood flowing into the heart collects in the atria. The right atrium fills with blood coming from the body; the left atrium fills with blood coming from the lungs.

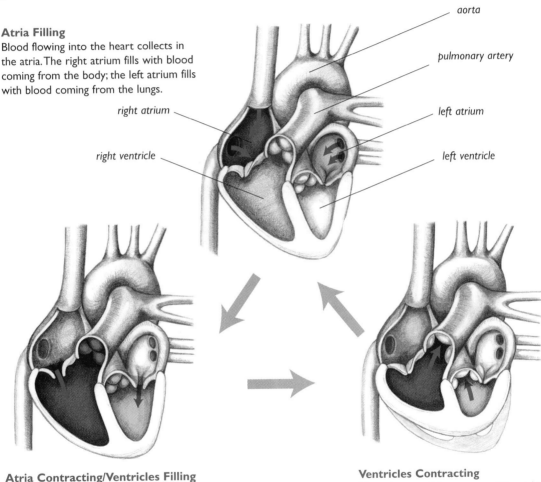

aorta

pulmonary artery

right atrium

left atrium

right ventricle

left ventricle

Atria Contracting/Ventricles Filling
When your heart beats, both atria contract, forcing blood into the ventricles.

Ventricles Contracting
Next, the ventricles contract. The right ventricle forces blood through the pulmonary artery to the lungs, where the blood will receive oxygen. The left ventricle pumps blood through the aorta, which carries the oxygenated blood throughout the body.

The heart beats according to an internal electrical charge that is created in special cells, called the *sinoatrial node,* located in the right atrium. When the sinoatrial node fires, it sends an electrical current through the heart muscle. This current signals the heart to beat. When the heart is working correctly, the heart beats in a regular rhythm. Irregular heartbeats, a "racing" heart, palpitations, or missed heartbeats can be caused by problems with the heart's electrical system.

What is blood pressure?

The force that is created by the heart pumping blood against the artery walls is called *blood pressure.* It is the combination of two measurements, systolic and diastolic. The top number, or *systolic pressure,* measures the force of the blood as it is pumped from the ventricles. The bottom number, or *diastolic pressure,* measures the force of blood against the walls of blood vessels while the heart is at rest. A normal blood pressure reading for an adult is less than 130/85. Lower readings are considered healthier. If your blood pressure is too high, your heart is working harder than it should, which can cause damage to the heart and blood vessels.

Blood Pressure Readings

	Systolic Pressure	Diastolic Pressure
Best	less than 110	less than 70
Normal	less than 130	less than 85
Borderline	130–139	85–89
Hypertension		
Stage 1	140–159	90–99
Stage 2	160–179	100–109
Stage 3	180–209	110–119
Stage 4	210 and above	120 and above

THE CIRCULATORY SYSTEM

The circulatory system is the network of blood vessels through which your blood travels to all parts of your body. The circulatory system includes arteries and arterioles (small arteries), which carry oxygen- and nutrient-rich blood from the heart to the rest of the body. It also includes veins and venules (small veins) that return blood to the heart from various parts of the body. Capillaries, which are very small blood vessels, connect arterioles to venules, so blood that has traveled from the heart to the body can begin the journey back to the heart and lungs.

You have roughly 5 quarts of blood in your body. It moves through the cardiovascular system at the rate of nearly 2,000 gallons a day—or roughly 2.5 ounces per heartbeat.

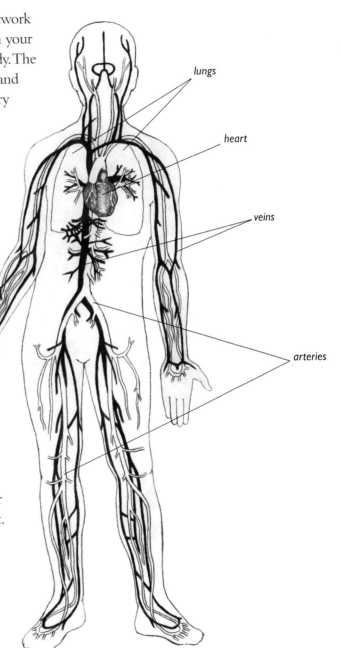

lungs

heart

veins

arteries

THE CORONARY ARTERIES

Like any other organ, the heart needs a constant supply of oxygen-and nutrient-rich blood to do its work. It receives this blood through the coronary arteries. The coronary arteries attach to the base of the aorta (where the aorta leaves the heart). Blood flows from the aorta, through the coronary arteries, and into the heart. The arteries go around the surface of the heart, branching off into smaller arteries that provide nutrients to different parts of the heart.

- **The left main coronary artery** is made up of two branches. The *left anterior descending* artery brings blood to the front of the heart; the *circumflex* brings blood to the left side and back of the heart.

- **The right coronary artery** brings blood to the right side and bottom of the heart. The *posterior descending branch* of the right coronary artery nourishes the back of the heart.

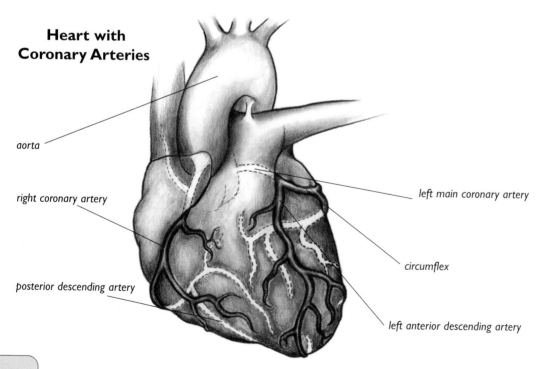

Heart with Coronary Arteries

aorta

right coronary artery

posterior descending artery

left main coronary artery

circumflex

left anterior descending artery

If the blood supply to any organ is disrupted or blocked, it can mean serious damage to that organ. The heart is no exception. This hardworking muscle needs oxygen and can be permanently damaged when supply is stopped.

The Heart Valves

The heart contains four one-way valves that keep your blood moving in the right direction as it goes through your heart. As blood is pumped through the heart and lungs, a valve opens to allow the blood to pass from one place to the next. Then the valve closes to keep the blood from moving backward.

Where are my heart valves and what do they do?

The four valves in the heart are:

- **The tricuspid valve,** between the right atrium and the right ventricle. This valve allows blood that has come from the body to move from its collecting place in the right atrium into the right ventricle, where it will be pumped on to the lungs.

- **The pulmonic valve,** between the right ventricle and the pulmonary artery. This valve opens with the squeeze of the right ventricle and sends the blood toward the lungs, where it will receive oxygen and nutrients.

- **The mitral valve,** between the left atrium and the left ventricle. This valve allows fresh blood that has returned to the heart from the lungs to move from its collecting place in the left atrium into the left ventricle, where it will be pumped to the rest of the body.

- **The aortic valve,** between the left ventricle and the aorta. This valve opens with the squeeze of the left ventricle and sends blood surging into the aorta, where it will start its journey to the rest of the body.

If the valves do not open properly, the heart has to push harder to force blood through them. If the valves do not close properly, blood can leak backward into its previous chamber, so there is not enough fresh blood being pumped into the arteries.

The Heart Valves

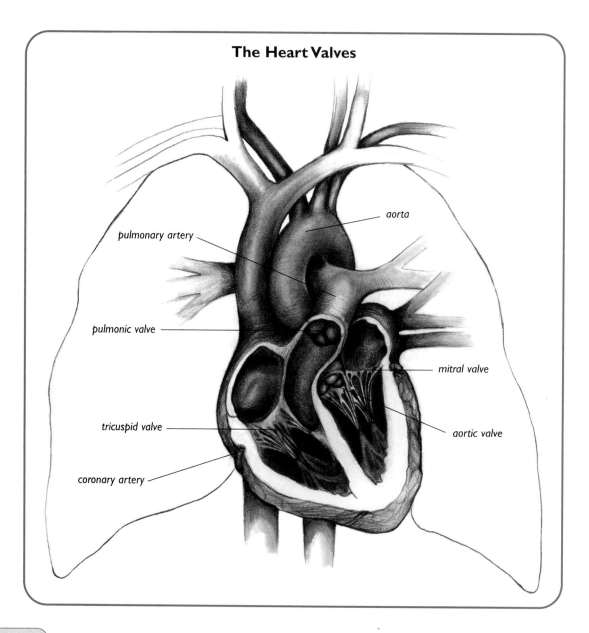

pulmonary artery

aorta

pulmonic valve

mitral valve

tricuspid valve

aortic valve

coronary artery

CHAPTER TWO

PROBLEMS WITH YOUR HEART

The heart is a marvelous and complex organ. When all is going well, we don't think much about our heart. But when something goes wrong, we may feel it in many ways—and not just in our chest. The heart's function affects every part of the body. Because the heart is so complex in its structure and operation, there are different kinds of problems that can occur.

Although heart problems can range from occasional irregular heartbeats to complete heart failure, we tend to worry about any problem with this essential organ.

In this chapter you will learn:

The symptoms of angina.

What "heart attack" means, and how to recognize one.

The symptoms of heart failure.

What happens when heart valves don't work right.

CORONARY ARTERY DISEASE

The coronary arteries bring oxygen and nutrients to your heart, so the heart can keep the rest of your body supplied with fresh blood. If these arteries become blocked, the heart gets less oxygen and cannot work efficiently.

The coronary arteries can become narrowed or blocked when fat and other materials build up in the arterial walls. This accumulation is called *plaque*. A narrowing of the arteries may occur anywhere in your body, but when it happens in the coronary arteries, it affects your heart's ability to function.

How serious is coronary artery disease?

According to the American Heart Association (AHA), coronary artery disease (also called coronary heart disease) caused 476,124 deaths in 1996 and is the single leading cause of death in America today. The AHA estimates that more than a million Americans will have a heart attack this year, and about one-third of them will die as a result.

Progression of Coronary Artery Disease

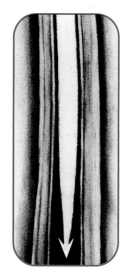
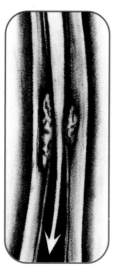
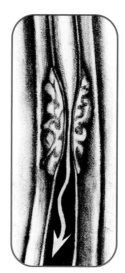
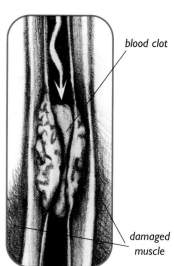

blood clot

damaged muscle

Healthy Coronary Artery

Plaque Build-Up

Angina

Heart Attack

The good news is that the rate of death from coronary artery disease has markedly declined since 1985, in part because people are more aware of how diet, exercise, and other lifestyle changes can reduce their risk, even after a heart attack.

Angina

It's estimated that more than 7 million people in the United States have angina. Angina is the name for chest pain that may result from coronary artery disease. It is not a disease, but a symptom of a disease. The correct medical name for the chest pain is *angina pectoris*. The name for the condition causing angina—in which the heart doesn't get enough blood and oxygen—is *myocardial ischemia*. It occurs when the coronary arteries are partially or fully blocked.

The first time you have an angina attack, you may think you are having a heart attack—or you may just think you ate the wrong food for lunch. If can be frightening: Perhaps you ran up the stairs a little faster than usual and now you feel a burning in your chest. Or you might feel queasy and very tired for a few minutes after an argument with your boss. If you have coronary artery disease, you may feel angina:

- When you exert yourself more than usual, whether exercising at the health club or running for the bus.

- When you are upset, angry, or feeling any other strong emotion.

- When you are eating, or just after eating.

- When the temperature is very hot or very cold.

Each of these situations puts extra stress on your heart and can cause angina.

Symptoms of angina may include:

- Unusual discomfort in the chest, arm, jaw, or back. This may be a sharp or dull pain, a burning sensation, or a feeling of tightness or pressure.

What are the symptoms of angina?

- Tingling, aching, or numbness in your arms, elbows, or wrists.

- Fatigue, queasiness, heavy sweating, shortness of breath, or indigestion.

An angina attack doesn't usually last more than a few minutes—generally less than 2 to 3—and the pain or discomfort will go away with rest or medication.

If you have an angina attack, stop and rest. If your doctor has pre-scribed nitroglycerin for you, sit down, put a tablet under your tongue, and let it dissolve. With rest and nitroglycerin, your angina should be gone within a couple of minutes. If it's not, take a second nitroglycerin tablet 5 minutes after the first. If you still feel angina, you can take a third tablet 5 minutes after the second. If your angina still hasn't gone away, call 911 for emergency help.

If you have never had an angina attack before, you should get emergency help when the symptoms first occur, even if they only last a few minutes. The symptoms of angina and a heart attack can be very similar, especially to someone who has never had either.

If you start having angina attacks more frequently, or if they seem to be lasting longer or getting more painful, notify your doctor. This can be a sign that you are developing a more serious heart problem.

Coronary Artery Spasm

If your angina occurs when you are at rest and not when you are unusually active, it may be the result of a coronary artery spasm. In this condition, one of the coronary arteries suddenly constricts, reducing or stopping blood to part of the heart. This can happen in a partially blocked coronary artery, but it may also occur in a normal coronary artery. The angina that occurs with a coronary artery spasm can be particularly painful, and it usually happens at night or in the early morning.

Although a coronary artery spasm can be very serious, it may be treated with medication.

Heart Attack

A heart attack, or myocardial infarction (MI), occurs when one of the coronary arteries is completely blocked: No blood is being supplied to the part of the heart served by that artery. Usually this happens when a blood clot enters a narrowed artery and completely blocks blood flow. When the artery is completely blocked and no blood is supplied to part of the heart, cells begin to die and permanent damage occurs. Occasionally the heart may be damaged by a coronary artery spasm.

The symptoms of a heart attack can be similar to those of angina. They include:

- A feeling of pressure, tightness, or squeezing pain in the center of the chest.

- Pain that spreads to the shoulders, neck, or arms.

- Lightheadedness or fainting.

- Sweating, especially "cold sweats."

- Queasiness or nausea.

- Shortness of breath.

- Sudden, intense anxiety.

- Unusual heartbeats, such as skipped beats or a series of very fast or very slow beats.

How will I know if I'm having a heart attack?

There is a difference between symptoms of a heart attack and those of angina: The symptoms do not go away with rest and they last more than a few minutes. A heart attack usually causes symptoms for more than 15 minutes. You may even have warning symptoms days or weeks in advance. The pain and discomfort may occur only in one part of your body, or it may move from one part to another (from you arm to your neck, for example). Or the pain may go away for a while and then reappear.

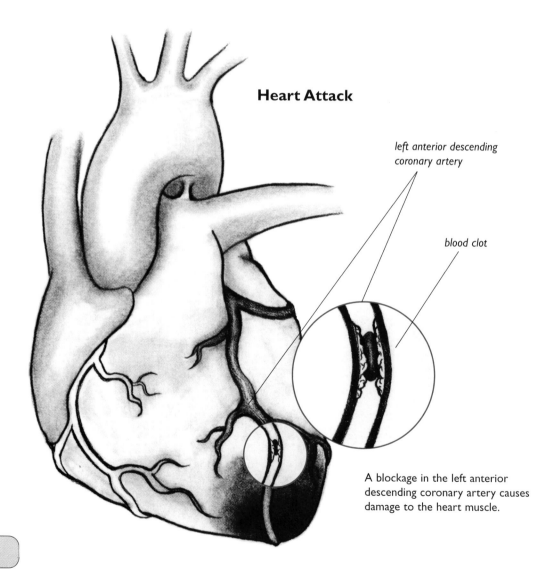

Heart Attack

left anterior descending coronary artery

blood clot

A blockage in the left anterior descending coronary artery causes damage to the heart muscle.

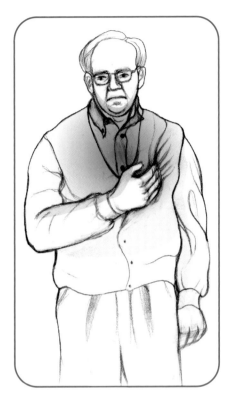

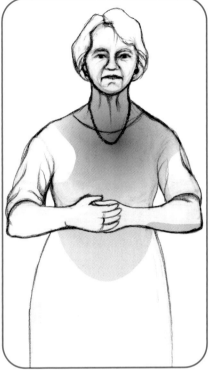

Are symptoms of a heart attack different for men and women?

For men, pain or tightness radiating from the chest is considered the "classic" symptom of a heart attack.

For women, the main symptoms may be nausea or shortness of breath. Many women do not experience pain or tightness in the chest when having a heart attack.

Pain or a tight feeling radiating from the chest are the "classic" symptoms of a heart attack. But other symptoms are common. For women, especially, the main symptoms of a heart attack may be shortness of breath or what seems to be an upset stomach. Elderly and diabetic people are also likely to have symptoms other than chest pain.

Don't let a "nonclassic" symptom cause you to postpone getting help for a heart attack. It's better to feel a little foolish because all you had was indigestion than to delay treatment for a heart attack.

According to the American Heart Association, about half the people who have heart attacks wait 2 hours or longer before calling for help. Most of the permanent damage done to the heart happens during the first hour after symptoms appear. If you wait too long to get help, serious damage to your heart is likely to occur.

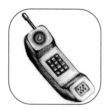

If you think you might be having a heart attack, don't wait to get help. Getting to a hospital quickly may reduce the amount of heart muscle damaged during the heart attack. Stopping the heart attack not only saves heart muscle, it reduces complications and the risk of dying. Once at the hospital, your condition can be diagnosed accurately. If a clot is blocking one of your coronary arteries, you may receive clot-dissolving medications or an emergency angioplasty, a procedure that opens blocked arteries (see chapter 5).

HEART FAILURE

Heart failure occurs when your heart can't supply enough blood to support the normal functions of your body. You can have mild heart failure with few symptoms, or severe heart failure with many symptoms. Heart failure can be caused by a number of different conditions, including:

- Coronary artery disease.

- A heart attack.

- High blood pressure.

- Valvular heart disease.

- An arrhythmia (abnormal heart rhythm).

- Chronic lung disease.

The symptoms of heart failure depend on which side of the heart has been affected. When failure occurs on the right side, blood doesn't pump to the lungs effectively. Instead, it backs up into the veins.

Symptoms of failure on the right side of the heart include:

- Swollen ankles or calves.

- A distended liver.

- Bloating in your abdomen.

- Lack of appetite.

- Nausea.

- Sudden weight gain.

- A need to urinate often during the night.

- Weakness.

What are the symptoms of heart failure?

If the left side of the heart is in failure, blood backs up into the lungs instead of being pumped to the rest of your body. There are two levels of symptoms for failure on the left side.

If heart failure is mild or moderate, symptoms can include:

- Shortness of breath at night or when you exercise.

- Fatigue.

- Insomnia.

- Rapid heart beat.

- Coughing or wheezing attacks.

If your heart failure is more severe:

- Fluid can leak into the air sacs of the lungs and cause coughing, severe shortness of breath, or a feeling of suffocation. If this occurs, seek medical attention immediately.

The treatment of heart failure depends on the cause of the heart failure and whether there was permanent damage to the heart. Valve disease can cause heart failure, for example, but surgery to repair the valve may allow your heart to operate normally again.

Cardiomyopathy

Cardiomyopathy is the deterioration of the heart muscle itself. There are three types of cardiomyopathy: dilated, hypertrophic, and restrictive. Each is a different kind of heart-muscle damage.

- **Dilated, or congestive, cardiomyopathy** is the most common form of cardiomyopathy. The heart becomes enlarged and, over time, less and less able to pump blood through the body the way it should. Because the heart is less efficient, it may pump harder, making the muscle even larger and more inefficient. You can have dilated cardiomyopathy for some time before you notice any symptoms. By the time it is diagnosed, the disease already may have reached an advanced stage.

- **Hypertrophic cardiomyopathy** is a rare form of heart disease in which the heart's muscle fibers are abnormal and the heart walls are too thick. This means there is less room inside the heart, so blood flow is obstructed. Usually hypertrophic cardiomyopathy is hereditary.

- **Restrictive cardiomyopathy** is usually the result of another disease elsewhere in the body that causes abnormal protein to come into the heart. As a result, the walls of the heart become stiff and inflexible, reducing blood flow. This is a rare form of heart disease.

Sometimes, the cause of cardiomyopathy is unclear. In other cases, cardiomyopathy can be caused by:

- Infection.

- Coronary artery disease.

- Thyroid disease or diabetes.

- Use of alcohol, some illegal drugs, or antidepressants.

- An inherited condition.

Symptoms of cardiomyopathy are like those of other heart failure, including:

- Difficulty breathing and shortness of breath.

- A dry, hacking cough.

- Difficulty sleeping, unless you are propped up.

- Swelling of the legs, ankles, and abdomen.

- Chest pain.

- An arrhythmia (abnormal heart rhythm).

- Heart palpitations.

- Nausea and vomiting.

- Decreased appetite.

- Sudden weight gain.

Cardiomyopathy can't be cured; once the heart muscle is damaged, it will remain damaged. Medications can help the heart pump more effectively and may reduce or ease symptoms of the disease. Some lifestyle changes—reducing stress or eliminating alcohol and drugs—may help slow the progress of the disease.

VALVULAR DISEASE

When they are working well, the four valves of your heart open and close completely. But a valve can be defective or become defective. Because each valve has a different location and function (see pages 9–10), a defect may have different symptoms.

Normal Valve

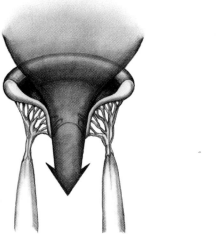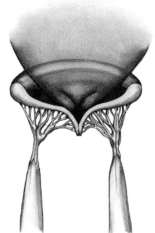

The heart valves open to let blood through, then close to prevent the blood from flowing backward.

The heart valves are:

- **The tricuspid valve,** between the right atrium and the right ventricle.

- **The pulmonic valve,** between the right ventricle and the pulmonary artery.

- **The mitral valve,** between the left atrium and the left ventricle.

- **The aortic valve,** between the left ventricle and the aorta.

The main causes of heart valve problems are:

- Congenital heart defects. Some babies are born with valves that do not open or close properly.

- Infections, such as bacterial endocarditis. Rheumatic fever is the infection that most often causes heart valve damage.

- Changes in the heart's structure caused by age.

Stenosis and Insufficiency

Damage to the heart valves can be described in two ways: *Stenosis* means that a valve can't open completely. Blood must be pumped through a smaller opening, so the heart must work harder. *Insufficiency* means that a valve doesn't close completely, so blood leaks back into the heart chamber from which it was pumped.

Stenosed Valve

Insufficient Valve

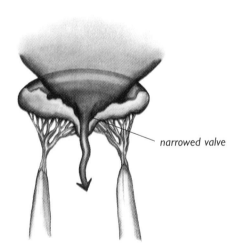
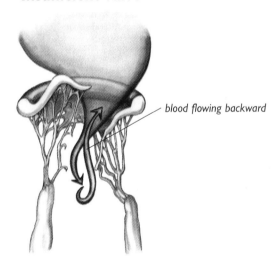

narrowed valve

blood flowing backward

In a stenosed valve, blood is pumped through a narrowed opening.

In an insufficient valve, blood leaks "backward" through the valve.

What happens
when heart valves
become defective?

If the valves in your heart aren't functioning properly, you may have changes in circulation, blood pressure, or heart rhythm. Without treatment, heart valve damage can lead to heart attack or heart failure.

Mitral Valve Stenosis and Mitral Insufficiency

Normally, blood pumping from the lungs to the heart collects in the left atrium, then moves through the mitral valve into the left ventricle. With mitral valve stenosis and mitral insufficiency, blood backs up into the left atrium instead of flowing easily into the left ventricle.

The symptoms of mitral valve stenosis and mitral insufficiency can include:

- An intense tired feeling.

- Shortness of breath.

- Coughing.

- A need to urinate often during the night.

- Heart murmur.

- Tenderness and swelling over the abdomen.

- Swelling in your legs and ankles.

- Difficulty sleeping unless your head is propped up.

- An irregular heartbeat that feels like a fluttering in the chest.

Aortic Valve Stenosis and Aortic Insufficiency

The aortic valve allows blood to be pumped from the left ventricle into the aorta, which carries blood to the rest of your body.

Problems with the aortic valve often cause symptoms similar to those of coronary artery disease. These may include:

- Fatigue.

- Chest pain.

- Shortness of breath when you exert yourself.

- A feeling of lightheadedness when you exert yourself.

- Heart murmur.

- Heavy sweating and flushed skin.

- Difficulty sleeping unless your head is propped up.

- A need to urinate often during the night.

- A faster heartbeat than usual, or occasional skipped beats.

Tricuspid Valve Stenosis and Tricuspid Insufficiency

The tricuspid valve allows blood to pump from the right atrium to the right ventricle. Damage to the tricuspid valve is less common than damage to the mitral or aortic valves. It may be caused by damage to other valves, or by disease of the heart muscle.

Symptoms of tricuspid valve stenosis and tricuspid insufficiency may include:

- Tenderness and swelling over the abdomen.

- Swelling in your legs and ankles.

- Extreme fatigue.

- A jaundiced, or yellow, color to your skin.

- Heart murmur.

- An enlarged liver.

Pulmonary Valve Stenosis and Pulmonary Insufficiency

The pulmonary valve, which allows blood to be pumped from the heart to the lungs, is seldom affected by disease, although it can be damaged by rheumatic fever. Adults rarely suffer damage to the pulmonary valve.

Mitral Valve Prolapse

About 5 percent of people in the United States have mitral valve prolapse, a heart condition that usually does not require treatment and poses little risk. This condition is sometimes called *the click-murmur syndrome* because of the sound that can be heard with a stethoscope.

Blood that has accumulated in the left atrium is pumped through the mitral valve into the left ventricle. From there, it pumps through the aortic valve into the aorta. When mitral valve prolapse occurs, the mitral valve "flops" or bulges backward into the left atrium as the left ventricle pumps blood through the aortic valve. This can sometimes cause mitral insufficiency (where the blood leaks back into the left atrium).

You may not be bothered at all by mitral valve prolapse, but some people have uncomfortable symptoms that can include:

- Heart palpitations, or a fluttery feeling in the chest.

- Chest pain.

- Fatigue or unusual nervousness.

- Shortness of breath.

- Anxiety.

Women are more likely than men to have mitral valve prolapse, and it is often hereditary.

For most people, no special treatment is necessary for mitral valve prolapse, but physicians may recommend reducing stress, cutting back on caffeine (which often reduces palpitations), or lying down with your feet raised to relieve chest pain. Physicians also may recommend the use of antibiotics before and after dental or surgical procedures.

Subacute Bacterial Endocarditis

Subacute bacterial endocarditis, also called SBE or endocarditis, is an infection of the inner lining of the heart and/or valves, caused by bacteria that have entered your heart. It is most likely to occur in people who have congenital heart defects or heart disease, or whose heart valves have been damaged or replaced. It is possible for someone with no previous heart disease to develop endocarditis, although this is uncommon.

If endocarditis worsens, bacteria can accumulate on the valves and then travel through the blood to other major organs, blocking blood flow and causing serious damage.

Symptoms of endocarditis may include:

- Chills and fever.

- Sweating, especially night sweats.

- Loss of appetite or weight loss.

- Headache.

- Fatigue and anemia.

- Joint pain.

- Heart murmur.

If you have a heart defect, have had valve replacement surgery, or have had endocarditis in the past, you need to take special care to avoid infections. Talk with your doctor about taking antibiotics before any medical treatment, including minor surgery or dental work.

OTHER CARDIOVASCULAR PROBLEMS

Arrhythmia

An arrhythmia is an abnormal heart rhythm—the heartbeat is too fast, too slow, or irregular. Normally, the heart beats because of an electrical impulse that originates in the *sinoatrial node* (special cells located in the right atrium). An arrhythmia usually occurs when the electrical impulse originates somewhere else in the heart.

For more information about heart rhythms, see chapter 6.

Thrombophlebitis

Thrombophlebitis is the development of a blood clot in the wall of a blood vessel, characterized by swelling around the clot. It can result from abnormal blood flow through the vessel. If untreated, part of a clot may eventually break away and travel through the body to the heart or lungs (called a *pulmonary embolism*), where it can cause serious damage.

How serious are blood clots?

Thrombophlebitis can develop under a number of circumstances—some you can change, some you can't. These include:

- Inactivity.

- A blow or fall that causes damage to the vessel.

- Intravenous drug use.

- Pregnancy.

- Obesity.

- Varicose veins.

- Congestive heart failure.

You are likely to feel symptoms of thrombophlebitis near the clot, usually in your arm or leg. These symptoms can include:

- Swelling of the arm or leg.

- Sensitivity to pressure.

- A visible red area along the vein.

- Headache.

- Fatigue.

- Fever.

Thrombophlebitis can be treated with surgery or another procedure to remove the clot, or medication to break up the clot.

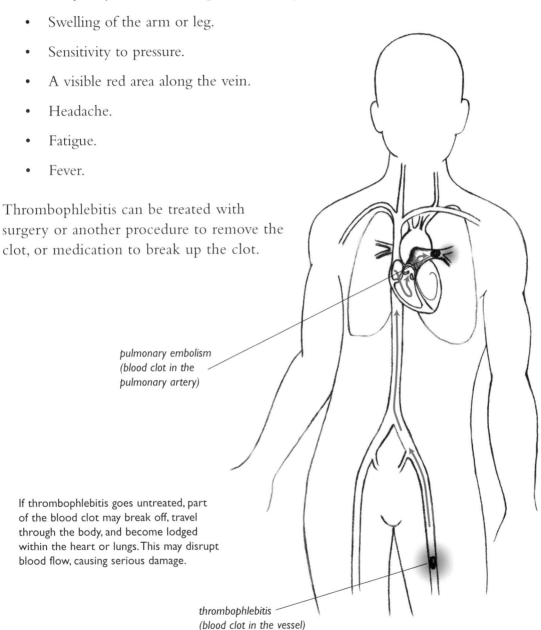

pulmonary embolism
(blood clot in the
pulmonary artery)

If thrombophlebitis goes untreated, part of the blood clot may break off, travel through the body, and become lodged within the heart or lungs. This may disrupt blood flow, causing serious damage.

thrombophlebitis
(blood clot in the vessel)

Aneurysm

An aneurysm occurs when the wall of an artery develops a weak spot that pushes outward when blood is pumped through it. The same thing can happen to the wall of one of the heart's chambers. Think of blowing up a long, thin balloon: As you blow harder, one spot that is a bit weaker than the rest of the balloon will suddenly bulge outward. This is similar to how an aneurysm occurs. If the aneurysm stretches the blood vessel too much, it can burst.

Aneurysms can occur in many parts of your body. Smoking, diabetes, high blood pressure, and high cholesterol increase the risk of an aneurysm. If you have high blood pressure, for example, the force of the blood pumping through your blood vessels is greater than normal. If there are weak spots in the artery walls, they may bulge with the increased pressure.

Ventricular Aneurysm

A ventricular aneurysm occurs on the left ventricular wall of the heart. It usually happens after a heart attack has caused a great deal of damage in that area. This condition may be treated surgically.

Aortic Aneurysm

Aortic aneurysms occur in the aorta, which is the largest blood vessel in your body. All of the blood pumped out of your heart must go through the aorta to get to the rest of your body.

Aortic aneurysms may form in the abdomen, near the kidneys, or in the chest. Because the aorta is your main artery, if an aneurysm in the aorta stretches to the point of bursting, it can be fatal.

A *dissecting aneurysm* occurs when the aorta wall separates into layers, causing blood to flow between the layers. This internal bleeding is very dangerous.

Usually you do not notice signs of an aneurysm until it begins to leak, grow, or dissect. If any of these things happen, you probably will feel pain around the area.

Some aneurysms cause symptoms that can include:

- Chest or back pain.

- Hoarseness, coughing, or shortness of breath.

- Problems swallowing.

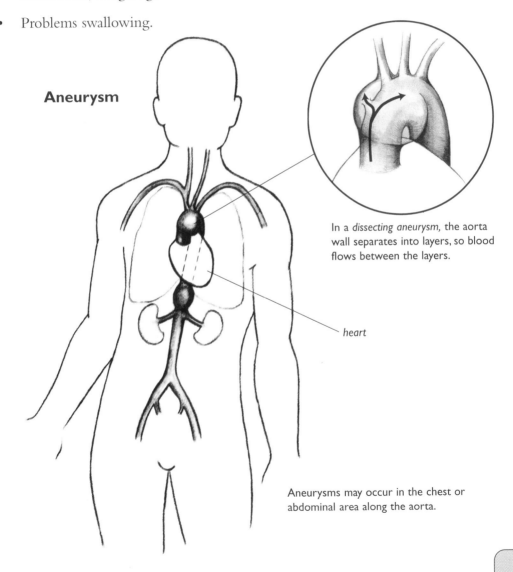

Aneurysm

In a *dissecting aneurysm,* the aorta wall separates into layers, so blood flows between the layers.

heart

Aneurysms may occur in the chest or abdominal area along the aorta.

An aneurysm may show up on a chest X-ray—in fact, that's how many people learn that they have one. It can be measured for size and location with magnetic resonance imaging (MRI) or computed tomography (CT) scanning.

If you have a small aneurysm, your physician may recommend regular exams and watching it for any change. If you have high blood pressure, medication may help reduce pressure on the aneurysm.

Large aneurysms and dissecting aneurysms must be treated right away, usually with surgery to replace the damaged section of the artery.

Pulmonary Hypertension

Pulmonary hypertension is high blood pressure in the blood vessels in your lungs. Clots may develop in these tiny blood vessels and increase the blood pressure even more. The cause of pulmonary hypertension is not known, but most people who develop it have a family history. Conditions that seem to be related to pulmonary hypertension include:

- Congenital heart disease.

- Collagen vascular disease.

- Severe viral illness.

- Blood clots in the lungs.

- Pregnancy.

- Birth control pills and some other drugs.

Pulmonary hypertension can happen at any age, but usually it happens to people who are 15 to 40 years old. Women are more likely to have pulmonary hypertension than men.

There is no cure for pulmonary hypertension, and the disease will progress, although usually slowly. Some people are helped by medication. Oxygen may be used to reduce pressure on the pulmonary artery.

Stroke

A stroke is a loss of blood to the brain that causes brain tissue to die. Narrowed arteries and high blood pressure, which are significant factors in heart disease, are also the major risk factors for stroke.

A stroke can be caused by insufficient blood flow due to narrowed arteries, an aneurysm, or a weakened blood vessel that bleeds into the brain. The effects of a stroke depend on which part of the brain is damaged. You may be weak or paralyzed on one side of your body, or you may be unable to speak normally.

The worst effects occur right after the stroke. Some of the brain cells die, but those that are only damaged often can recover functioning.

CHAPTER THREE

RISK FACTORS

If you have heart disease, one of the first things you may ask is, "Why me?" A number of things—from your family's health history to your lifestyle—can affect your chances of having heart disease. These are called "risk factors." When a medical provider takes your history, it's important to tell the truth about risk factors because they can affect your care.

Some risk factors can be changed—for example, you can always stop smoking or enjoy a healthier diet. When risk factors cannot be changed, like age or gender, you can still reduce your risk of heart disease by changing your lifestyle.

In this chapter you will learn:

How family history affects your risk of cardiovascular disease.

That heart disease is a problem for both men and women.

How you can control the three major risk factors: smoking, cholesterol, and hypertension.

How lifestyle affects heart disease.

RISK FACTORS YOU CAN CHANGE

Smoking

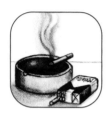

A U.S. Surgeon General has called smoking "the most important of the known modifiable risk factors for coronary heart disease in the United States."

This means that of all the risk factors you can change, smoking is the most important. Even if smoking is your only risk factor, it is a very serious one. And combined with other risk factors, it seems to greatly increase your chances of developing cardiovascular disease. For example:

- Although oral contraceptives alone may not increase your risk of heart disease, if you smoke and take oral contraceptives, your risk of heart disease is even greater than the risk caused only by smoking.

- If you have a family history of heart disease and you smoke, your risk of heart disease is greatly increased.

The number of cigarettes you smoke matters. Smoking one pack of cigarettes a day doubles your risk of heart disease; smoking two packs quadruples your risk.

How does smoking affect heart disease?

The nicotine in cigarettes causes your heart to beat faster, increasing your body's need for oxygen. At the same time, the carbon monoxide from cigarettes reduces the amount of oxygen your red blood cells can carry. The combined effect of nicotine and carbon monoxide means that your heart needs more oxygen, but gets less. This contributes to the development of heart disease.

If you don't smoke, but you are surrounded by smokers at home or elsewhere, you still may be at a higher risk. Secondhand smoke contributes to the development of heart disease.

Cholesterol

When you have your cholesterol checked, you will usually be told your total blood cholesterol level. A total cholesterol level of less than 200 is considered best. If your cholesterol level is 200 to 239, you are on the borderline of high cholesterol. A reading of 240 or more means you have high cholesterol and a substantial risk of developing heart disease.

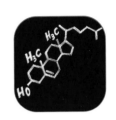

Cholesterol is a fatty substance found in all of your body's cells and in your blood. It is needed to build tissues, cell membranes, hormones, and bile. Cholesterol is made in the liver and released into your blood, where it is carried to other parts of the body.

What is cholesterol?

There are several types of cholesterol. *Low-density lipoprotein (LDL),* is often referred to as "bad cholesterol" because a higher level of LDL increases your risk of heart disease. Normal levels of LDL are below 130.

High-density lipoprotein (HDL), is often referred to as "good cholesterol" because higher levels of HDL are associated with a reduced risk of heart disease. Normal HDL levels are above 35.

Triglycerides are the fats carried by cholesterol. An elevated level of triglycerides is associated with a higher risk of heart disease. A normal triglyceride level is less than 200.

You should discuss your cholesterol levels with your healthcare provider. He or she will help you determine what your risk is and how you can change your diet and lifestyle to help change your cholesterol levels. Although a tendency toward high cholesterol levels may be inherited, it is possible to maintain a lower level through medication or careful diet.

High Blood Pressure

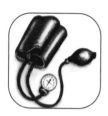

High blood pressure, or hypertension, is itself a cardiovascular disease. It means that your heart has to pump harder than it should to get blood through your body. If your heart is pumping harder, both it and your arteries are strained. If your heart pumps harder for a long time, it may get larger, making it even more difficult to pump well.

With high blood pressure, your arteries and arterioles may become narrow and less flexible. Although this happens to some degree as you get older, high blood pressure causes it to happen at an earlier age—and at a faster pace.

High blood pressure means that you are at greater risk for other cardiovascular disease, including blood clots, heart attack, and heart failure.

Hypertension is sometimes called "the silent killer" because it is such a significant factor in heart disease and other organ failure. Ninety to ninety-five percent of the time, the cause of high blood pressure is unknown. For most people, high blood pressure can be controlled by diet, exercise, and medication.

Sedentary Lifestyle

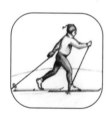

If you don't exercise regularly (that is, an average of 30 to 60 minutes, 4 to 6 times a week), you are more likely to develop cardiovascular disease.

Most adults exercise a little, but not often enough and not hard enough. A stroll through your neighborhood on a Sunday afternoon may be better than no activity at all, but to get real benefits from exercise you need to do it regularly and it needs to increase your heart rate. While exercising, you should be working somewhat hard. Generally, you will feel as if you are breathing faster and deeper than when you started. Your doctor may tell you to aim for a certain heart rate while exercising.

If you have symptoms of heart disease and have had a sedentary lifestyle (you haven't exercised enough) up until now, consult your medical care providers before starting an exercise program. Trying to do too much too fast can be harmful for some people with cardio-vascular disease. For more information on exercise, see chapter 7.

Weight

Even if weight is your only risk factor, it is a significant one. If you are overweight, you are at greater risk of developing heart disease, and it will be more difficult for you to control it. If you are obese, the extra weight puts a strain on your heart, aggravates high blood pressure and high cholesterol levels, and increases your risk of devel-oping Type 2 diabetes—all risk factors for heart disease.

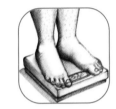

Being obese does not mean being a little overweight; if you are carrying "an extra 5 pounds," you probably shouldn't worry about your weight.

To determine whether your weight puts you at greater risk for heart disease, don't just look at the number on your scale—look at the shape of your body. If you have gained most of your weight around your waist and belly, you are at greater risk. You can assess whether you are overweight and at greater risk of heart disease in two ways:

1. **The waist-to-hip ratio** is just that, a measurement of your waist, divided by the measurement of your hips. Your waist should be smaller than your hips, meaning that your waist-to-hip ratio should be less than 1. For men, a healthy waist-to-hip ratio is less than 0.9. For women it's less than 0.8. To take your waist-to-hip ratio accurately, you should:

- Stand straight, with your feet together. Measure your natural waist using a cloth measuring tape, and don't suck in your breath or pull the tape tight. Write down the measurement to the nearest inch (not 31.5 inches, but 32 inches, for example).

- Measure the widest part of your hips and rear. Again, don't pull the tape too tight, and measure to the nearest inch.

- Divide the first measurement by the second.

2. The body mass index (BMI) is a rough measure of your body fat. The National Institutes of Health have developed guidelines for determining obesity based on the idea of BMI. Obesity is defined as a BMI of 30.0 or higher. Overweight is defined as a BMI of 25.0 to 29.9.

The formula for determining BMI is a bit complicated. It's based on dividing your height in inches by your weight, but there are a few other steps. The chart on the following page does the math for you. To find your BMI:

- Use a good scale on a flat surface. Take off your shoes, and wear as little clothing as possible. (The scale in your doctor's office should be accurate.) Write down your weight to the nearest pound.

- Get an accurate reading of your height. If you are at your doctor's office, you can ask to be measured there. At home, stand against a wall and make sure your shoulders, rear end, and head are touching the wall. Ask someone to use a ruler to mark the spot on the wall that reflects the highest point on your head. Then measure from the floor to the mark, and write down your height to the nearest inch.

- Use the table on the following page to determine your BMI.

Body Mass Index Table *(for adults only)*

HEIGHT	60"	62"	64"	66"	68"	70"	72"	74"	76"	78"	80"
WEIGHT											
100	20	18	17	16	15	14	14	13	12	12	11
105	21	19	18	17	16	15	14	14	13	12	12
110	22	20	19	18	17	16	15	14	13	13	12
115	23	21	20	19	18	17	16	15	14	13	13
120	23	22	21	19	18	17	16	15	14	14	13
125	24	23	22	20	19	18	17	16	15	14	14
130	25	24	22	21	20	19	18	17	16	15	14
135	26	25	23	22	21	19	18	17	16	16	15
140	27	26	24	23	21	20	19	18	17	16	15
145	28	27	25	23	22	21	20	19	18	17	16
150	29	27	26	24	23	22	20	19	18	17	17
155	30	28	27	25	24	22	21	20	19	18	17
160	31	29	28	26	24	23	22	21	20	19	18
165	32	30	28	27	25	24	22	21	20	19	18
170	33	31	29	27	26	24	23	22	21	20	19
175	34	32	30	28	27	25	24	23	21	20	19
180	35	33	31	29	27	26	24	23	22	21	20
185	36	34	32	30	28	27	25	24	23	21	20
190	37	35	33	31	29	27	26	24	23	22	21
195	38	36	34	32	30	28	27	25	24	23	21
200	39	37	34	32	30	29	27	26	24	23	22
205	40	38	35	33	31	29	28	26	25	24	23
210	41	38	36	34	32	30	29	27	26	24	23
215	42	39	37	35	33	31	29	28	26	25	24
220	43	40	38	36	34	32	30	28	27	25	24
225	44	41	39	36	34	32	30	29	27	26	25
230	45	42	40	37	35	33	31	30	28	27	25
235	46	43	40	38	36	34	32	30	29	27	26
240	47	44	41	39	37	35	33	31	29	28	26
245	48	45	42	40	37	35	33	32	30	28	27
250	49	46	43	40	38	36	34	32	30	29	28
255	50	47	44	41	39	37	35	33	31	30	28
260	51	48	45	42	40	37	35	33	32	30	29
265	52	49	46	43	40	38	36	34	32	31	29
270	53	49	46	44	41	39	37	35	33	31	30
275	54	50	47	44	42	40	37	35	34	32	30
280	55	51	48	45	43	40	38	36	34	32	31
285	56	52	49	46	43	41	39	37	35	33	31
290	57	53	50	47	44	42	39	37	35	34	32
295	58	54	51	48	45	42	40	38	36	34	32
300	59	55	52	49	46	43	41	39	37	35	33

U.S. National Institutes of Health

It may not seem easy, but you *can* take off weight—and greatly reduce your risk of heart disease. As with some of the other risk factors, regular exercise and a healthy diet can work wonders.

If you have heart disease, do not start any kind of diet and exercise program without consulting your healthcare team, and do not take any kind of weight reduction medication unless it is under your physician's care. While the benefits of losing weight are considerable, trying to do it too fast can put too great a strain on your heart and other organs.

Stress

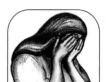

People sometimes joke about being a "Type A" personality, someone who is always under stress. But stress is no joke for your heart.

Stress causes physical reactions in your body. If you are anxious about how to pay the bills this month, or angry at your partner, or feeling threatened by a new boss at work, your body will react. Your heart rate may increase, your blood pressure may rise, blood vessels might constrict, more blood may flow to your brain.

These physical responses to stress helped our Stone Age ancestors to escape danger or kill food for their families. But in the modern world, stress seems to be there all the time, not just when the saber-toothed tiger is about to attack, and its effects can add to the risk of heart disease. If you already have heart disease, stress may trigger heart pain and increase your chances of having a heart attack.

Some stress is unavoidable. Money problems, illness, family disagreements, a deadline at work . . . these are a part of our lives. You can't always change stressful situations, but you can change the way you react to stress. For example, your job may be very stressful, but if you feel good about the work you do, you may experience less stress.

Often when we get angry or upset in a stressful situation, we have talked ourselves into these emotions. "This is awful," we say to ourselves. "It shouldn't be like this. What a terrible thing. I can't stand for it to be this way." While this seems like a normal reaction—and it is a common reaction—there are other ways to think about a stressful situation. "I don't like this, but I'm not going to let it upset me," you might say to yourself. "It isn't fair, but I know I will get through it." You might want to talk to a counselor or therapist to help you develop different ways of responding to stress in your life.

Some stress can be controlled. If you always feel rushed, ask yourself why. Do you tend to forget how much time it will take to get somewhere, so you're constantly on the verge of being late? If so, leave earlier. Are you booked every night of the week? Schedule some "down time" for yourself—and stick to the schedule. Only you can pinpoint the origins of your stress, but it's worth taking an inventory to see if you can make changes. To help reduce stress:

- **Spend time with friends and family.** Being with people you enjoy is a wonderful stress reducer.

- **Exercise regularly.** Besides being good for your body, exercise helps you calm down.

- **Get enough sleep.** If you have problems sleeping when you're stressed, talk to your doctor about ways to encourage sleep.

- **Keep your home and work areas organized,** so you don't get stressed trying to find things you need.

- **Give yourself more time when you're working on a project,** whether cleaning the house, writing a school paper, or preparing a presentation for your boss.

- **Find something that makes you feel peaceful.** Maybe it's a hot bath, maybe pleasant music, maybe a favorite scent.

Diabetes

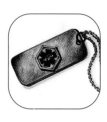

Nearly 9 million Americans have diabetes, and more than 600,000 new cases are diagnosed each year.

When we say "diabetes," we mean the disease *diabetes mellitus,* which is the body's inability to make or use insulin the way it should. Insulin, a hormone made in the pancreas, controls the amount of sugar in the blood and the way sugar is used in the body's cells.

Type-1 diabetes, or insulin-dependent diabetes, usually occurs before the person is 30 years old. In fact, this is often called "child-onset" diabetes because most people who have it developed it in childhood. In Type-1 diabetes, the pancreas does not produce enough insulin. People with Type-1 diabetes have such a serious lack of insulin that they must take manufactured insulin for the rest of their lives.

Type-2 diabetes, or noninsulin-dependent diabetes, usually occurs after age 40. About three-quarters of the people who have Type-2 diabetes are overweight. With Type-2 diabetes, the pancreas is producing insulin, but the person's body has become resistant to the insulin. Type-2 diabetes can be controlled through diet, exercise, and medication.

There is no cure for diabetes, only control. If you have diabetes it will affect your treatment for heart disease.

Uncontrolled diabetes is a significant risk factor for coronary artery disease, but even mild or well-controlled diabetes can contribute to heart attacks or reduced blood circulation to the heart. Maintaining healthy blood sugar levels will reduce these risks and limit the serious effects of diabetes.

Hormones

Changes in hormone levels can affect your risk of heart disease. For women, estrogen seems to help prevent heart disease before menopause. When menopause occurs, hormone levels drop and the risk of heart disease tends to increase. Few women under 40 develop heart disease, but the risk increases between the ages of 40 and 65. In fact, about half of heart attack victims 65 and older are women.

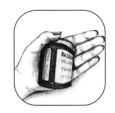

There has been some concern about whether oral contraceptives (birth control pills) increase the risk of cardiovascular disease. Early studies showed that women taking birth control pills were more likely to develop heart disease. However, recent research indicates that the newer forms of oral contraceptives, which have smaller amounts of estrogen, show no significant increase in risk—as long as other risk factors are controlled.

Many women use hormone replacement therapy (HRT) to ease some of the problems associated with menopause and to reduce the loss of bone density that sometimes comes with age. Perhaps the most important benefit of HRT is that it may help prevent heart disease.

Research shows that HRT increases HDL cholesterol (the "good" cholesterol) and lowers LDL cholesterol (the "bad" cholesterol). It seems to help increase blood flow and keep the arteries flexible.

There is some concern about whether HRT increases the risk of cancer. Women with a family history of breast cancer should discuss this risk with their healthcare providers.

Alcohol

Whether to drink alcohol—and how much to drink if you do—has been a subject of debate. One day you read an article in the newspaper that says you should have a glass of red wine every day to protect against heart disease; a week later you read that alcohol can

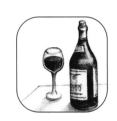

contribute to heart disease. A friend tells you that vinegar will have the same effect as alcohol. Your uncle says that it's red wine that helps your heart, no other kind of alcohol.

Will alcohol decrease my risk of heart disease?

Research shows that drinking a little alcohol may help protect against heart disease. Alcohol seems to raise the "good" cholesterol and reduce the "bad" cholesterol in the blood. A little, or moderate, drinking is defined by the American Heart Association as 1 ounce of alcohol a day: one mixed drink, one glass of wine, or two beers. Drinking more than this amount doesn't increase your protection against heart disease; in fact, it can increase the risk.

Heavy drinking, whether done regularly or in "binges," increases stress on the heart. It can contribute to heart diseases ranging from cardiomyopathy (an enlarged heart) to arrhythmias (irregular heartbeats).

There is a slightly increased risk of heart disease for people who drink no alcohol, but this doesn't mean you should start drinking. Alcohol abuse is a serious problem in itself.

RISK FACTORS YOU CAN'T CHANGE

Family History

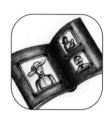

If someone in your close family—a parent, grandparent, brother, or sister—has had cardiovascular disease, you run a greater risk of getting it yourself.

The age at which your relative developed heart disease is important. If a relative developed or died of heart disease at a fairly late age (70 or older), your risk is not much greater than that of someone who had no relatives with heart disease. If a relative had heart disease before age 55, your risk of heart disease increases. If more than one family member has had early heart or circulatory disease (before age 55), you are at an even greater risk.

Because you can't change your family history—or any inherited tendency toward heart or circulatory disease—it's even more important that you maintain a healthy lifestyle.

Race and Ethnic Background

Although family history is more likely to predict your risk of heart disease than race or ethnic background, race and ethnicity are still considered risk factors.

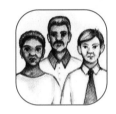

African Americans are more likely to have high blood pressure than other racial populations. High blood pressure is linked to other cardiovascular problems, including blood clots, heart attack, and heart failure. For African Americans, the rate of heart disease—and the rate of death from heart disease—is higher than that of any other group in the United States.

If you are African American, know your risks. Find out if your family has a history of heart disease, and maintain a healthy lifestyle.

Gender

For many years heart disease—particularly the heart attack—was mainly thought to be a problem for men. Until recently, little research was done on how women develop heart disease.

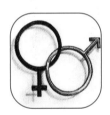

Most women are more afraid of breast cancer than heart disease, but heart disease is far more common: More than 20 percent of women in the United States have some form of cardiovascular disease.

Up until menopause, usually around age 50, women have a lower rate of heart disease than men. Once they reach menopause, however, their estrogen level drops—and their risk of heart disease increases. By age 65, men and women are about equally likely to have a heart attack.

Women with heart disease tend to have more serious complications than men. They are more likely to die if they have a heart attack, and they don't do as well after surgery. (Remember that these are overall findings taken from individual experiences; they don't predict how you will do if you have a heart attack or heart surgery.) No one knows for certain why women with heart disease tend to have more problems than men, but doctors and researchers have some theories:

Why do women seem to have more problems with heart disease than men?

- **Age may be a factor.** Women are likely to be older when they have a heart attack. This may make them more vulnerable not only to the effects of the heart attack, but also to problems during and after surgery.

- **For some treatments, such as coronary artery bypass surgery, smaller people do less well than larger people.** Women are often smaller than men, so that may explain why they don't do as well in surgery.

- **For women, the symptoms of heart disease may not be "typical" symptoms.** For example, a man having a heart attack may experience chest pain, whereas a woman may experience fatigue and sense that something is wrong. Chest pain may or may not occur. For this reason, women—and sometimes doctors—may not recognize the symptoms for what they are.

- **Many women ignore the symptoms of heart disease,** because they do not think it is likely to happen to them. Some conditions get worse if they are not treated in the early stages.

- **More women than men have diabetes, a major risk factor for heart disease.** Furthermore, diabetes seems to have a greater effect on heart disease in women than in men. If a woman with diabetes has a heart attack, she is more likely to have a second heart attack than a man with diabetes.

Heart disease in women sometimes goes undetected until it becomes a serious problem. Remember, for women, the symptoms of a heart attack may or may not involve chest pain.

You should be alert to the following heart attack symptoms:

- Chest discomfort, including pressure, tightness, pain, or indigestion.

- Pain in the neck, shoulder, jaw, or upper abdomen.

- Shortness of breath.

- Fatigue.

- Nausea.

- A sense that "something just isn't right."

Age

Heart disease happens to people of all ages. Younger people with heart disease often have a family history of early death from heart attack or other cardiovascular problems. Some have a genetic or congenital (from birth) heart defect that goes undetected for many years but at some point begins to cause problems.

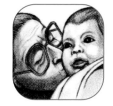

Younger people with several risk factors—diabetes, too much weight, lack of activity, overuse of alcohol, smoking—may develop heart disease at an earlier age.

If you are a man under age 45, or a woman under age 55, you are not at great risk of developing heart disease—in the absence of other risk factors. When you reach age 45 or 55, the risk increases with each year.

In most cases, younger people are more successful in controlling their heart disease than older people, if they follow their medical team's instructions and reduce any risk factors in their life.

CHAPTER FOUR

FIGURING OUT WHAT'S WRONG

When medical providers try to figure out just what your symptoms mean, it can be pretty intimidating. They may use a variety of equipment and tests with difficult names.

The tests used to diagnose heart disease are very sophisticated. Physicians can look right inside your arteries to find out if there are blockages—and they can pinpoint just where the blockages are. They can use radiation to highlight areas of the heart, and a computer to "map" your heart's structure. Or they may simply have you walk on a treadmill while they measure your heart response.

In this chapter you will learn:

What electrocardiograms and echocardiograms are.

How a catheter is used to look at your heart.

How a computer image of your heart is created.

How radioactive materials can show your heart's blood flow.

ELECTROCARDIOGRAM

If you have any symptoms of heart disease, the first thing your doctor is likely to do is an electrocardiogram, usually called an EKG or ECG. This is a fairly simple measure of the electrical activity of the heart. It shows whether your heart is functioning normally or whether it seems to be damaged or having problems.

On pages 94–95 you will find an example of an image produced by an EKG. You are probably already familiar with this image—it's the one displayed on the heart monitors shown on television and in the movies.

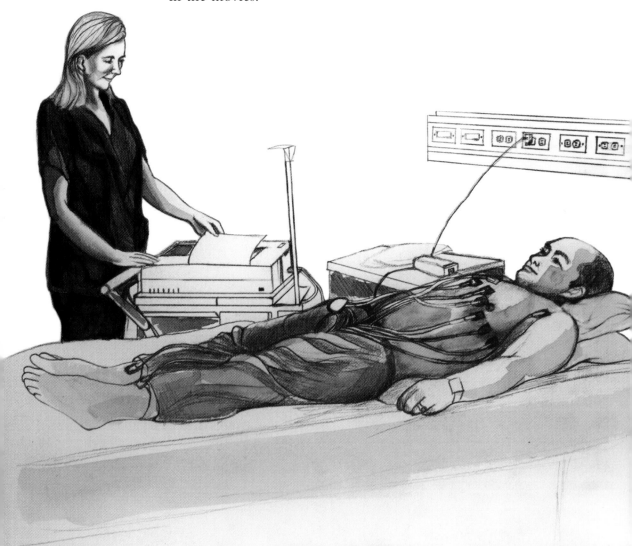

The electrocardiogram itself doesn't take very long—generally less than 5 minutes—but when used as part of a stress test, it will take more time.

- You will be asked to take off your clothing from the waist up. Women may leave their brassiere on.

- Electrodes will be placed on your wrists and ankles and across your chest. Each electrode has a harmless gel applied to it, which helps conduct electrical signals from your heart to the electrocardiogram machine.

- Wires connect the electrodes to the machine, which records the electrical signals from the heart. Each signal gives a slightly different look at the way your heart is functioning.

An electrocardiogram may be performed in a variety of ways. If it is done with a stress test, you will walk on a treadmill as electrodes conduct electrical signals from your heart to the electrocardiogram machine. This will show how your heart performs under stress.

If you have occasional symptoms of heart rhythm problems, you might have an ambulatory electrocardiogram (Holter monitor). In this test, you wear a small, battery-powered device that monitors your heart rhythm as you go about your normal life for 24 hours. If you have any symptoms, you write them down. Your doctor can use the electrocardiogram results and your notes about symptoms to identify any irregularities.

Some electrocardiograms transmit readings over the phone. If you begin to have symptoms of a heart irregularity, your hospital or doctor can see it right away, even if you are at home when the symptoms occur.

ECHOCARDIOGRAM

An echocardiogram might sound more familiar if you think of it as an ultrasound. Perhaps when you or someone you love was pregnant, an ultrasound test was done so you could see the baby in the womb. An echocardiogram uses ultrasound waves to look at the heart and to show its operation on a television screen. Like the electrocardiogram, an echocardiogram examines the heart without anything being inserted into the body.

- You will be asked to take off your clothing from the waist up and put on a hospital gown.

- The technician will look at your heart while you are resting. As you lie on an examining table, a small device lubricated with a harmless gel will be put on your chest. The technician will move the device slowly around your chest to see the heart from different positions.

- You can see the images of your heart on a television screen. It also will be recorded on videotape.

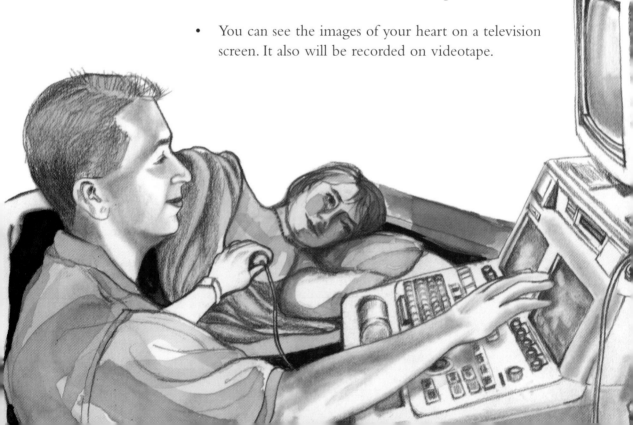

- An electrocardiogram will be done along with the echocardiogram. By looking at images from both the electrocardiogram and echocardiogram, your doctor will have a better sense of how your heart is working.

Transesophageal Echocardiography (TEE)

A transesophageal echocardiogram is a way to get a better echocardiogram image of your heart by recording the image from inside your esophagus. Your esophagus—which you may know better as your food pipe—is just behind your heart. An echocardiogram image made from inside the esophagus can give a more accurate look at your heart than an echocardiogram made from outside your chest.

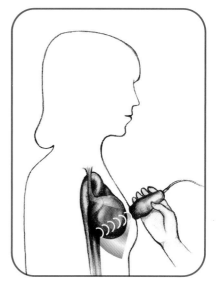

An echocardiogram uses sound waves to look at the heart, much like an ultrasound is used to see a baby inside the mother's womb.

A transesophageal echocardiogram is safer and less difficult than it may sound. Your throat will be treated with an anesthetic so it will be numb as the tube is inserted, and you may be given a sedative to help you relax.

If you stay relaxed during the procedure, it will be easier for you. Try to stay calm, breathe easily, and think about relaxing things.

- For a transesophageal echocardiogram, your doctor will have you lie on your left side.

- Your doctor will put a flexible tube into your mouth and then down into your esophagus. A small probe at the end of the tube makes sound waves that can be seen on a monitor while the doctor moves the probe into different positions.

Is a TEE painful?

- You may feel the probe as your doctor moves it, but you shouldn't feel any pain.

- The test will take 20 to 40 minutes as your doctor looks at different images of your heart.

- After the test you may have a bit of scratchiness in your throat. Treat it the way you would any sore throat, with cold drinks and cough drops or hard candies. (Bleeding, a stiff neck, or pain deep in your esophagus is not normal, so tell your doctor right away if you experience any of these.)

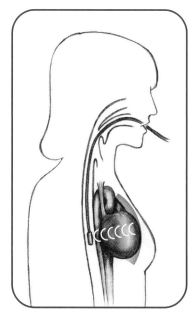

A transesophageal echocardiogram uses sound waves from inside the esophagus to create an image of the heart.

- Be sure your throat is no longer numb before you eat or drink anything.

STRESS TESTS

Because the heart works differently when it is under stress, looking at your heart while you are at rest only gives part of the picture. Many problems can be diagnosed better if your doctor looks at your heart's functioning both at rest and after stress. There are two types of stress tests: exercise and nonexercise.

Exercise Stress Tests

When your doctor wants to look at your heart while it's under stress, you may be asked to take a stress test. An exercise stress test is used to determine your heart's response to physical activity. You will get on a treadmill or an exercise bike and walk or pedal until you reach your target heart rate or until symptoms occur.

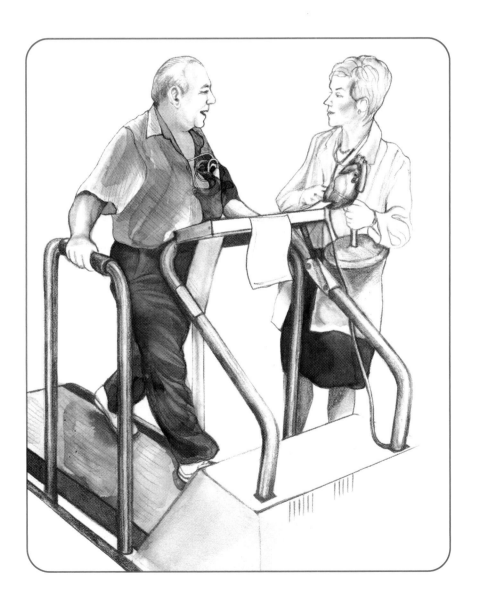

Is there any danger in taking a stress test?

If you have angina, or chest pain, you may worry that an exercise stress test will be dangerous or cause greater pain. But exercise stress tests have been given for many years, and problems are very rare. You will be closely monitored the whole time, and your doctor or technician will stop the test if you are short of breath, dizzy, suddenly tired, or feeling pain.

To monitor changes in your heart's electrical activity, an electrocardiogram will be used before, during, and after the exercise stress test. A stress test usually takes 30 to 45 minutes, but the imaging procedure done with it may take several hours.

There are two kinds of stress tests: a stress echocardiogram and cardiac nuclear imaging.

Stress Echocardiogram

A stress echocardiogram looks at your heart while you are at rest and again after you have exercised.

- Your doctor or technician will perform an echocardiogram.

- After images are taken of your heart at rest, you will be asked to exercise, usually on a treadmill or stationary bicycle.

- You will be expected to exercise until your heart is beating rapidly, or until you develop symptoms.

- A second set of images is taken after you finish exercising. Your doctor can compare the way your heart works when you are resting with the way it works after activity.

A stress echocardiogram is a safe, noninvasive, relatively simple way for your doctor to assess heart problems.

Cardiac Nuclear Imaging

Using a gamma camera, your doctor can make a nuclear image that will show how blood flows through your heart. This kind of test is sometimes used if you have chest pain and your doctor doesn't know what is causing it. It's also used to see if surgery has helped the flow of blood through your heart. Your doctor may refer to nuclear imaging as a thallium or Cardiolite test.

You will be injected with a small amount of radioactive material (thallium or Cardiolite), which will be absorbed by your heart. The radiation is less than what you might get from having X-rays.

> Is it dangerous to receive a radioactive injection?

The parts of your heart that have the strongest blood flow will absorb the most radioactive material. When the heart is scanned, your doctor will be able to see which parts of your heart may have low blood flow.

Nuclear imaging may be done when you are at rest or when you are exercising on a treadmill. It takes about 3 hours for the entire test. About 30 to 45 minutes of this will be scanning time.

- For a resting scan, a technologist will inject you with a small amount of thallium. After you wait about 15 to 30 minutes, the technologist will take images of your heart with the gamma camera. You will need to stay very still while the scanning is done.

- If you are having an exercise test, you will first have a resting scan, then you will get on a treadmill. Your doctor will monitor your heart while you walk on the treadmill, and will increase the speed and incline of the treadmill. When the doctor feels your heart is beating more strongly, Cardiolite will be injected through an intravenous line. You'll keep walking on the treadmill with the IV in your arm.

- If the doctor asks for a stress test and you aren't able to exercise on a treadmill, medication (Persantine, adenosine, or dobutamine) may be used to increase your heart rate, giving the effect of exercise. Cardiolite will be injected for the scan.

- In either case, a second scan of your heart will be made 30 to 60 minutes after the first scan.

- The doctor who conducts the test will talk to your doctor, who will discuss the results with you.

To prepare for nuclear imaging:

- Don't eat or drink anything for 4 hours before the exam.

- Don't have caffeine (coffee, tea, chocolate, or certain soft drinks) for 24 hours before the exam.

- People with diabetes should not take take oral medications before the test, unless their doctor has told them to. Those on insulin should talk to their doctor about reducing their dose.

Nonexercise Stress Tests

If you can't exercise, your doctor may use a drug to stimulate your heart in order to see how it functions under stress.

Stress Echocardiogram with Dobutamine

Dobutamine will be given slowly through an IV line in your arm. For a few minutes after the drug has been given, you will feel your heart pound. This is exactly what your doctor wants—it allows the doctor to see your heart while it's stressed. As your heart rate increases, an echocardiogram will be done so your doctor can see if the stress causes any changes in your heart. Continuous electrocardiogram monitoring will be done throughout the test.

Nuclear Imaging with Persantine, Adenosine, or Dobutamine

Nuclear imaging allows your doctor to see how blood flows through your heart. This test is sometimes used if you have chest pain and your doctor doesn't know why. It may also be used to show how the heart's blood supply has improved after surgery or other treatment.

- The doctor will first perform this test while your heart is at rest. A technologist will inject you with a small amount of radioactive material (such as thallium or Cardiolite). The radiation from this material is less than you might get from having X-rays. You will wait about 15 to 30 minutes, then the technologist will take images of your heart with a gamma camera. You will need to stay very still while the scanning is done.

- If the doctor wants to see your heart under stress, and you aren't able to exercise on a treadmill, medication (Persantine, adenosine, or dobutamine) may be given through an IV. The medication will make your heart beat faster, as if you were exercising.

- The technologist will again inject you with small amounts of radioactive material. The radioactive material will help show how blood flows through your heart. A special camera will display images of your heart. These images will also be stored on computer disk.

- After you have rested for a while, your doctor will do another nuclear scan to see if there are signs of narrow arteries or heart muscle damage.

CORONARY ANGIOGRAPHY

A coronary angiogram, or arteriograph, is an X-ray of your heart. It allows your doctor to check for coronary artery disease, heart valve problems, heart abnormalities, or an aneurysm. A coronary angiogram is often performed along with an angioplasty (described in chapter 5). The procedure takes place in the hospital, but unless you are already a patient in the hospital, you will not need to stay overnight to have the test done. The procedure should last between 30 to 60 minutes.

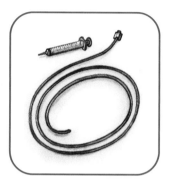

Catheter tube used in a coronary angiogram.

- Before the doctor can X-ray your heart, a dye must be injected into the coronary arteries. To do this, your doctor will insert a thin catheter into an artery in your arm or groin, then thread it carefully into the aorta. Once in the aorta, the doctor will move the catheter into the coronary arteries—the arteries that supply the heart with the blood and oxygen it needs to work properly. The doctor is able to see where the catheter is going by looking on a monitor.

- When the catheter is in place, the doctor will use it to inject dye into your coronary arteries. Now the X-ray camera will be able to see your coronary arteries as well as the smaller blood vessels branching off from them. The doctor may move you, or the whole examining table, in order to get X-ray pictures from different angles.

Will I be awake during an angiogram?

- You will be awake during the angiogram, and the idea of having a tube inserted into your heart may make you nervous. Your doctor may give you a sedative before the examination so you will be calm during the procedure.

- You will be given a local anesthetic, so you won't feel pain when the catheter is inserted. Most people don't feel pain during the procedure, but there may be some minor discomfort.

- When the catheter is in place and the dye is released into the coronary arteries, you may feel warm or flushed for 20 to 30 seconds. Most people feel some sense of heat; this is normal and is not dangerous.

- A few people have some chest pain after the procedure, but it eases quickly.

- Some people are allergic to the kind of dye used in the angiogram. If you have allergies or asthma, let your doctor know before the examination.

- You will need to lie flat for several hours after the procedure, as directed by your doctor.

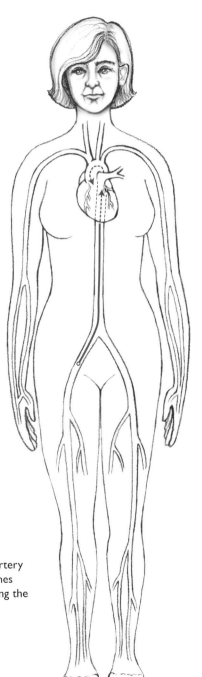

With a coronary angiogram, the doctor inserts a catheter through an artery in the arm or groin, then threads it carefully into the aorta until it reaches the coronary arteries. Dye is injected into the coronary arteries, allowing the doctor to check for abnormalities.

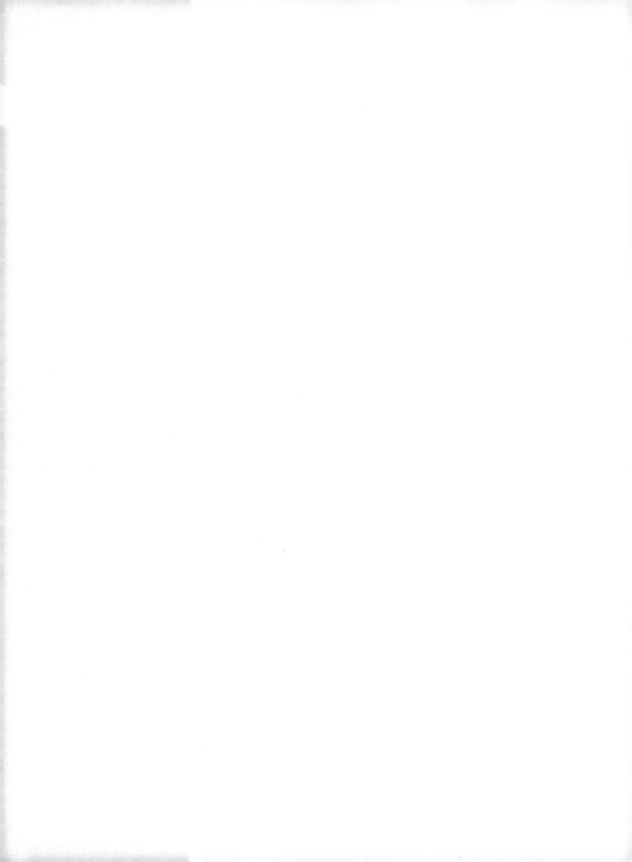

TREATMENTS

Treatments for heart problems range from the very simple—changes in lifestyle, perhaps coupled with medication—to the dramatic, such as heart transplant surgery.

Some treatments, such as the pacemaker, have proved successful for many patients over several decades. Newer treatments show signs of one day providing relief for people with very serious heart disease. New treatments, and new ways of using standard treatments, are constantly being developed.

In this chapter you will learn:

Descriptions of common medications for heart disease.

When "invasive" interventions are used.

What a coronary bypass is.

How defective valves can be repaired or replaced.

New areas of research.

MEDICATION

For many heart problems, medication will be the first treatment your doctor recommends. There are medications that can help regulate your heart rate, prevent blood clots, control chest pain, and lower cholesterol. Even if you undergo other treatments for your heart problem, such as a pacemaker or coronary bypass surgery, medication is likely to be a permanent part of your therapy.

- Learn the names of your medications, what they look like, and the reason you are taking them. If you're confused, ask your doctor or pharmacist about your medications.

- Understand the directions for each medication.

- Know which medications you're allergic to, and keep a list of your allergies and current medications in your wallet or purse.

- Get prescriptions refilled 5 to 7 days before you run out.

- Store your medications—in their original containers—in a cool, dry place away from bright light.

- Don't stop taking a medication without talking with your doctor.

- Don't take medications in the dark—it's too easy to make a mistake.

- If you miss more than two doses of a medication, call your doctor.

- Before you have surgery, dental work, emergency treatment, or other medical care, tell your doctor or dentist which medications you are taking.

If you have trouble remembering to take your pills, talk to your doctor about the best way to schedule them during the day. You might try a daily medication dispenser, a special pill box with different compartments for different times of the day. Or you might photocopy the medication schedule on the following page.

How can I keep track of my medications?

Researchers are developing new and more effective medications for heart disease all the time. Some of these medications are described on the pages that follow.

ACE Inhibitors

Angiotensin-converting enzyme (ACE) inhibitors are drugs that block the production of a natural substance that narrows blood vessels. This lowers your blood pressure and relaxes your blood vessels so your heart doesn't have to pump as hard. The result is improved circulation throughout your body. ACE inhibitors include:

- **Enalapril (Vasotec),** which may cause low blood pressure, dizziness, fainting, lightheadedness, persistent dry cough, or a rash. This medication also can cause high levels of potassium in the blood, which can lead to an irregular heart rate, numbness, tingling, and nervousness.

- **Captopril (Capoten),** which also helps decrease kidney damage in people with diabetes. Possible side effects include low blood pressure, lightheadedness, rash, cough, decreased sense of taste, dizziness, stomach upset, swelling of the face, and swelling inside the mouth and throat.

- **Lisinopril (Zestril, Prinivil),** which also helps decrease kidney damage in people with diabetes. Possible side effects include low blood pressure, lightheadedness, rash, cough, decreased sense of taste, dizziness, stomach upset, swelling of the face, and swelling inside the mouth and throat.

Medication Chart

MEDICATION NAME:	Morning	Afternoon	Evening	Night
Dose: Directions:	Comments:			

MEDICATION NAME:	Morning	Afternoon	Evening	Night
Dose: Directions:	Comments:			

MEDICATION NAME:	Morning	Afternoon	Evening	Night
Dose: Directions:	Comments:			

MEDICATION NAME:	Morning	Afternoon	Evening	Night
Dose: Directions:	Comments:			

MEDICATION NAME:	Morning	Afternoon	Evening	Night
Dose: Directions:	Comments:			

MEDICATION NAME:	Morning	Afternoon	Evening	Night
Dose: Directions:	Comments:			

Antiarrhythmics

There are a number of medications used to control different kinds of arrhythmias. See chapter 6 for information about these medications.

Antiplatelets

Antiplatelet medications, such as clopidogrel (Plavix) or aspirin, help prevent blood clots from forming. This reduces the chance of a heart attack or stroke, which can happen when a blood vessel is blocked by a blood clot. If you have a stent (described later in this chapter), you need to take an antiplatelet medication to make sure clots don't form around the stent.

- **You should not take antiplatelet medications if you have certain medical conditions,** including stomach problems, a blood disorder, serious bleeding, or liver problems.

- **You should not take antiplatelet medications if you are pregnant or breastfeeding.**

- **Your doctor needs to know what other medications you are taking before prescribing antiplatelets.** This is especially important if you take aspirin, digoxin (Lanoxin), seizure medications, theophylline (Theo-Dur), cimetidine (Tagamet), or warfarin (Coumadin).

- **Antiplatelets should be taken with food or after meals.**

- **Possible side effects** include rash, diarrhea, gas, stomach upset, nausea, and mild stomach pain. If you have fever, chills, sore throat, cough, unusual bruising or bleeding, yellowing of the skin or eyes, dark urine, bloody or dark bowel movements, or severe stomach pain, call you doctor as soon as possible.

- **Do not take two doses at once.** If you miss a dose, take it as soon as you remember. If it is close to time for the next dose, skip the missed dose and take the next dose at your regular time. (For example, if you are to take the medication every 6 hours, and you missed a dose 4 hours ago, then wait 2 hours until it's time for the next dose.)

Beta-Blockers

Beta-blockers, such as atenolol (Tenormin), metoprolol (Lopressor), nadolol (Corgard), and propranolol (Inderal), slow your heart rate and reduce blood pressure. They may be used to prevent angina, or chest pain. In low doses, beta-blockers have few side effects.

- **Take beta-blockers exactly as prescribed by your doctor.** Do not stop without checking with your doctor. If you miss a dose, take it as soon as possible—unless you're within 8 hours of the next dose. Never take a double dose.

- **If you are taking an extended-release form of a beta-blocker, you must swallow the tablet or capsule whole.**

- **Possible side effects** include impotence, dizziness, light-headedness, drowsiness, sleeping problems, anxiety, nervousness, constipation, diarrhea, nausea, and vomiting.

- **Call your doctor if you have** depression, confusion, skin rash, unusual bleeding, angina, back or joint pain, shortness of breath, slow heart rate, or swollen ankles, feet, or lower legs.

- **Beta-blockers make you more sensitive to cold** because they tend to decrease the blood supply to your skin, fingers, and toes.

Calcium Channel Blockers

Calcium channel blockers, like diltiazem (Cardizem) or verapamil, are used to prevent or reduce angina, or chest pain. They also help reduce high blood pressure. These medications relax blood vessels, increasing the amount of blood that flows into the heart and making it easier for the heart to work.

- **Sustained-release capsules must be swallowed whole.** Don't break, crush, or chew them.

- **Side effects** may include dizziness or lightheadedness, weakness, heartburn, nausea, and headaches. If you have irregular heartbeats, shortness of breath, constipation, or swelling of the feet or hands, tell your doctor.

- **Check your pulse before taking the medication.** If your pulse is slower than normal or less than 50 beats per minute, talk to your doctor before taking another dose.

- **Call your doctor immediately if** your hands, face, lips, eyes, throat, or tongue swell, or if you have trouble swallowing or breathing.

- **Do not take two doses at once.** If you miss a dose, take it as soon as you remember. If it is halfway until time for the next dose, skip the missed dose and take the next dose at your regular time.

Diuretics

Diuretics, such as furosemide (Lasix) and torsemide (Demadex), reduce blood pressure and decrease swelling caused by excess water in the body. Reducing the amount of water in the body also reduces the volume of the blood and relaxes the artery walls. This means your heart doesn't have to work as hard to pump blood to the rest of your body.

The biggest concern about many diuretics is that they reduce potassium in your body, which can lead to thirst, cramps, irregular heart rate, mood changes, nausea, or vomiting.

- **To reduce the danger of potassium loss, eat potassium-rich foods,** including bananas, oranges and other citrus fruits, apricots, and dates. Your doctor also may prescribe a potassium supplement.

- **Do not take two doses at once.** If you miss a dose, take it as soon as you remember, unless it's close to time for the next dose.

Nitrates or Nitroglycerin

How fast does nitroglycerin work?

Nitroglycerin is a very common treatment for angina, or chest pain. It can be taken as soon as the pain occurs and usually brings relief within a few minutes.

Nitroglycerin dilates (expands) the walls of your blood vessels. Angina occurs when your heart must pump harder to push blood through narrowed arteries. When the nitroglycerin takes effect, the arteries dilate so your heart doesn't have to work as hard.

- **When you experience angina, or if you're about to do something that normally causes you chest pain, put a tablet of nitroglycerin under your tongue and let it dissolve.** Don't swallow the nitroglycerin. If you are using nitroglycerin spray, spray into your mouth.

- **Sit down while you're taking nitroglycerin.** You may get dizzy or lightheaded.

- **If you still feel discomfort, take a second nitroglycerin tablet 5 minutes after taking the first.**

- **If there is still discomfort, you can take a third nitroglycerin tablet 5 minutes after taking the second.**

- **If you still feel discomfort after taking three nitroglycerin tablets, you should call 911 for emergency help.** Do not drive yourself to the hospital or doctor's office.

- **Keep the nitroglycerin with you at all times.**

- **Don't store your nitroglycerin with other pills or with cotton;** these can absorb the nitroglycerin vapors and make it lose strength.

- **Keep nitroglycerin tablets in the bottle they came in.** Replace the tablets every 6 months.

Your doctor may prescribe long-acting nitrates, which you take several times during the day in order to prevent angina. Long-acting nitrates can become less effective if taken all the time, so your doctor may recommend waiting 8 to 12 hours between doses. Besides long-acting pills, nitroglycerin patches and ointments are available for long-term treatment.

Headaches are a common side effect of nitroglycerin. Drinking alcohol is likely to increase any headaches or dizziness caused by nitroglycerin.

Thrombolytics

Thrombolytic drugs, like Activase (tPA) or Retavase (rPA), are used to quickly dissolve a blood clot that has blocked a coronary artery and is causing a heart attack. The drug binds to the blood clot and begins to dissolve it right away. The sooner the drug is given, the sooner the clot is dissolved so that blood can flow to the heart again. If the drug is given quickly enough, less permanent damage is likely to occur.

Thrombolytic drugs are given in the hospital or emergency room. Although these drugs may successfully dissolve the blood clot causing your heart attack, you will likely need other therapy for your heart disease, such as medication, surgery, or a revascularization procedure.

The greatest risk in taking a thrombolytic drug is that bleeding may occur somewhere else in the body. Some minor bleeding is expected, but your doctor and medical team will watch for signs of internal bleeding.

REVASCULARIZATION PROCEDURES

Revascularization is a procedure used to open up narrowed arteries. If you have coronary artery disease, and your arteries have become narrow with an accumulation of plaque, your doctor may recommend a revascularization procedure. A stent (described later in this chapter) will likely be implanted during the procedure.

Angioplasty

What is balloon angioplasty?

Angioplasty (PTCA) is often done along with an angiogram (described in chapter 4). You remain awake during the procedure, although you may be given a sedative to help you relax. You may have heard angioplasty referred to as "balloon angioplasty" because a small balloon is used to reopen the artery. Here's how an angioplasty works:

- Your doctor will first perform an angiogram. You will be given a local anesthetic, usually in the groin, where a catheter will be inserted into a blood vessel and threaded up into your heart. A dye is injected through this catheter so your doctor can see the narrowed artery on a fluoroscope, a special X-ray machine.

- To perform the angioplasty, your doctor will use the puncture made during the angiogram, threading a guiding catheter through the blood vessel until it reaches the narrowed artery.

Balloon Angioplasty

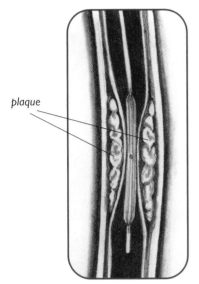

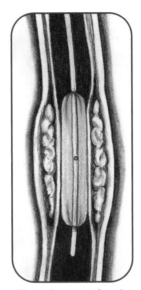

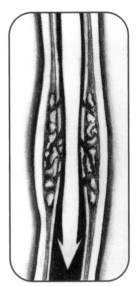

plaque

A balloon catheter is placed in the narrowest part of the artery.

The balloon is inflated, compressing the plaque into the artery wall.

The newly opened artery allows blood to flow more freely to the heart.

- Next, a second catheter—called a "balloon catheter" because it has a balloon near its tip—is threaded through the guiding catheter. The balloon is placed in the narrow part of the artery.

- The balloon is inflated for a minute or so, then deflated. As the balloon expands, it presses the plaque into the artery wall, opening the artery and letting blood flow more freely to the heart. The balloon may need to be inflated several times in order to compress the plaque against the artery wall. You may feel some chest pain each time the balloon is inflated. Your doctor can give you pain medication if you need it.

- Finally, the balloon is deflated and both catheters are removed.

After an angioplasty, you may have no more blockage in that artery. However, in 30 to 40 percent of patients, the blockage returns. To prevent this, your doctor may recommend implanting a stent during the procedure (described on the following page).

Coronary Extraction Atherectomy or Rotablator Procedure

In some cases, doctors prefer to remove the plaque clogging an artery, rather than compress it into the artery wall. This can be done with an atherectomy or a Rotablator procedure, where the plaque is scraped or ground away using a special kind of catheter.

As in balloon angioplasty, a hollow catheter is threaded into your heart, then a second catheter (either an atherectomy catheter or Rotablator) is inserted into the first catheter.

Atherectomy or Rotablator Procedure

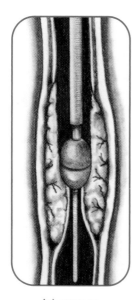 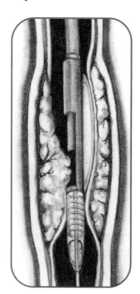 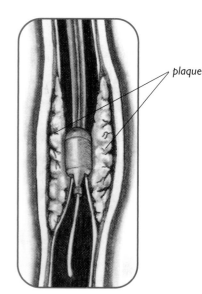

plaque

Atherectomy   Extraction Atherectomy   Rotablator Procedure

The atherectomy catheter has a blade on one side that scrapes or shaves the plaque from your artery wall. When in place, the blade rotates to shave the plaque, which collects in the catheter tip. The catheter may have a balloon that presses the blade against the blockage so the doctor can scrape the plaque more effectively.

With *extraction atherectomy,* a rotating blade at the tip of the catheter shaves the plaque, while a vacuum pulls the pieces of plaque into the catheter and out of your body.

A *Rotablator* has a football-shaped "burr" at the top with a diamond covering. When the catheter is inserted into the narrowed part of the artery, the burr rotates and grinds the plaque. With a Rotablator, the pieces of plaque ground from the wall are too small to be harmful. They are swept away by your bloodstream.

If you have no complications, you may be able to do many of your normal activities within a few days after an atherectomy, but you should check with your doctor first.

The affected artery may get clogged with plaque again, and your symptoms may return. Be sure to tell your doctor if you notice increased angina, an irregular heart rate, or any other symptom of coronary artery disease.

Stent

A coronary stent is a tube of metal mesh—usually stainless steel—that is sometimes implanted in your artery during one of the revascularization procedures described in previous pages. The stent helps keep the artery open.

- First, the artery is opened through balloon angioplasty, an atherectomy, or a Rotablator procedure.

- A catheter, with the compressed stent on top of a balloon, is threaded through the artery to the blockage.

- The balloon is then inflated, expanding and opening the stent. The expanded stent helps make sure the artery is open.

- Once the stent is open, the balloon is deflated and removed, leaving the stent in place. The stent will eventually become part of the artery wall.

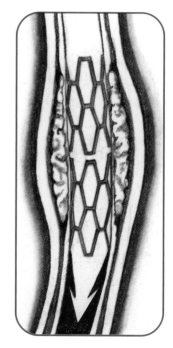

With a stent in place, blood flows more freely through the artery.

Sometimes, more than one stent is needed to keep a longer section of the artery open. The doctor will place the stents one at a time.

A stent reduces the chance that an artery will become narrow again after a revascularization procedure. However, because it is a foreign object placed permanently in your body, there can be some complications. You will be given medication to keep your blood flowing freely, so clots won't form around the stent after it is first implanted.

You will be given a stent-patient identification card, which you should keep with you at all times. If you need emergency medical attention, those who are treating you should know that you have an implanted stent.

If you have symptoms of angina, call your doctor right away.

SURGERY

Coronary Bypass

In the last 20 to 30 years, coronary bypass surgery has become a common treatment for diseased coronary arteries. You probably have heard friends or acquaintances talk casually about "my triple bypass" or "my quadruple bypass." If your doctor recommends bypass surgery to restore blood flow to your heart, your chances of having successful surgery—and of feeling much better afterward—are excellent.

Bypass surgery does just that: It bypasses a blockage in the artery, creating a new path for blood to flow to your heart. The surgeon will use a section of an "extra" blood vessel from somewhere else in your body, (usually a vein from your leg, or an artery from your arm or from inside your chest wall), to create a bypass around the blocked part of the artery. During bypass surgery the doctor could make more than one bypass, depending on the number and location of blockages.

This is major surgery. The risks include:

- Breathing problems during or after surgery.

- Bleeding.

- Infection.

- Injury to nerves during surgery.

- Heart attack or stroke.

How risky is bypass surgery?

Operating on the heart is complicated because the heart is always in motion. Some surgeons will perform a bypass while the heart is beating. (See "Surgery on the Beating Heart" later in this section). More likely, you will be connected to a heart-lung machine that will deliver oxygen to your blood and circulate blood throughout your body, so your heart can be stopped while the bypass is made. When the surgery is finished, your heart will be restarted.

The Surgery

This is what may happen during your bypass surgery, which probably will take from 4 to 6 hours:

- You will be given a general anesthetic, so you will be asleep during the surgery.

- The surgeon will make an incision down the middle of your chest and separate your breastbone, so the heart can be worked on. (Once the heart surgery is done, the breastbone will be put back together with stainless steel wires and should heal in 6 to 8 weeks.)

- Tubes will connect your heart to the heart-lung machine. Your heart will be stopped and the heart-lung machine will take over, supplying your blood with oxygen and pumping blood through your body.

- When your heart is still, the surgeon will make an incision in your arm, leg, or chest, removing part of a blood vessel to use for the bypass. Blood flow in your body will not be significantly affected by the removal of one or more of these vessels.

- Very carefully, with tiny stitches, the surgeon will sew one end of the blood vessel to a spot just below the blockage in your coronary artery. The other end of the vessel will be sewn onto the aorta. Now, blood flowing from the aorta into the coronary artery will no longer be blocked; it will have a new path in the bypass graft.

- If more than one coronary artery is blocked, the surgeon may do several bypasses.

Coronary Bypass

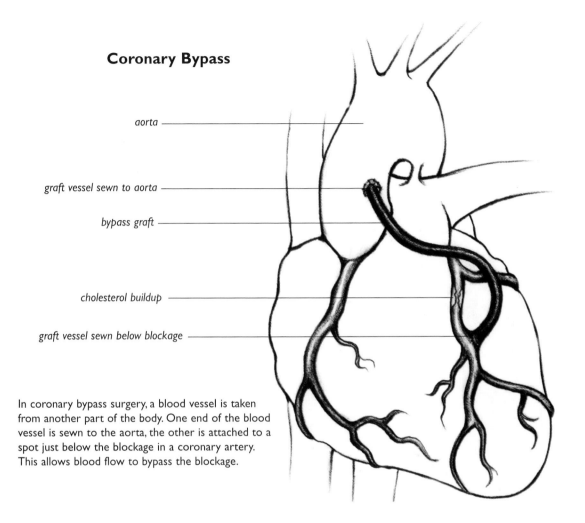

aorta

graft vessel sewn to aorta

bypass graft

cholesterol buildup

graft vessel sewn below blockage

In coronary bypass surgery, a blood vessel is taken from another part of the body. One end of the blood vessel is sewn to the aorta, the other is attached to a spot just below the blockage in a coronary artery. This allows blood flow to bypass the blockage.

- The surgical team will restart your heart. When it is beating successfully, you will be disconnected from the heart–lung machine. The surgeon will wire your breastbone together and sew up the chest incision.

- You will be taken to the Intensive Care Unit (ICU), where you will be monitored. You will have a breathing tube in your throat, drainage tubes, a bladder catheter to drain your urine, IV lines, and lines connecting you to a heart monitor.

Recovery

Recovery time after bypass surgery varies from one person to the next. It is not uncommon for a patient to stand up and take a few steps within 24 hours after surgery. As you begin to recover, you will be disconnected from various tubes and then moved to a cardiac unit until you are ready to go home. Your doctor will talk with you about how long you need to stay in the hospital and what kind of in-hospital rehabilitation you will have.

It may take at least 6 to 8 weeks before you can return to all of your normal activities. For some people, the improved blood flow makes them feel so much better that they can actually do more than they could before their surgery. Others will feel weakened by the surgery for several months. Do not push yourself too hard or too quickly.

Follow your doctor's instructions carefully after you return home, and be sure to take the medications prescribed for you on a regular schedule. For more information on recovering after surgery, see chapter 7.

Surgery on the Beating Heart

Although it is still common to use the heart-lung machine during coronary bypass surgery, some doctors are now doing surgery on hearts that are still beating. In one kind of surgery, the doctor makes an incision in the chest over the blocked coronary artery. The doctor then detaches a blood vessel from the leg, arm, or chest wall and uses it to bypass the blockage.

If surgery is done without stopping the heart, it can shorten the patient's time in the hospital, reduce the stress and pain caused by traditional surgery, and speed recovery. However, many doctors consider this kind of surgery experimental. Also, it isn't appropriate for every patient.

Heart Valve Surgery

Heart valves that are stenotic (unable to open properly) or inefficient (unable to close properly) sometimes can be corrected through surgery. A surgeon might repair your heart valve or replace it.

Some replacement valves are made of metal or plastic, some come from donors (people who have died), and some come from pigs or cows.

Repairing or replacing a heart valve is considered major surgery. The risks include:

- Breathing problems during or after surgery.

- Bleeding.

- Infection.

- Injury to nerves during surgery.

- Heart attack or stroke.

Mechanical valves are made of metal or other materials, so they last a long time. However, because these materials aren't normally found inside the human body, blood clots may form around them. If you have a mechanical valve, you will have to take anticlotting medication for the rest of your life.

Tissue valves from humans, pigs, or cows are more easily accepted by the body, but they are not as durable, and they may be damaged while waiting to be transplanted. Tissue valves are chemically treated to prevent animal cells and bacteria from being transmitted to the recipient.

Can tissue valves transmit diseases or bacteria?

Operating on the heart is complicated because the heart is always in motion. During the surgery, you will be connected to a heart-lung machine that will deliver oxygen to your blood and circulate blood throughout your body, so your heart can be stopped while the valve repair or replacement is made. When the surgery is finished, your heart will be restarted.

The Surgery

This is what will happen during your valve surgery, which probably will take from 4 to 6 hours:

- You will be given a general anesthetic, so you will be asleep during the surgery.

- The surgeon will make an incision down the middle of your chest and separate your breastbone, so the heart can be worked on. (Once the heart surgery is done, the breastbone will be put back together with stainless steel wires and should heal in 6 to 8 weeks.)

- Tubes will connect your heart to the heart-lung machine. Your heart will be stopped and the heart-lung machine will take over, supplying your blood with oxygen and pumping blood through your body.

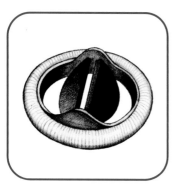

Mechanical valves are made of metal or other materials, so they last longer than tissue valves. Recipients of mechanical valves must take anticlotting medication for the rest of their lives to prevent blood from clotting around the valve.

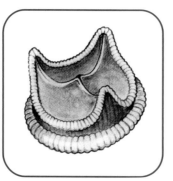

Tissue valves come from cows, pigs, or human donors. They are chemically treated to prevent the transmission of disease.

- The surgeon will make an incision in your heart or aorta to reach the valve.

- If the valve is to be repaired, the surgeon may cut and separate parts of the valve that won't open fully, or shorten and tighten parts of the valve that won't close properly. This kind of repair is done with very tiny surgical stitches.

- If the valve is to be replaced, the surgeon will cut out part or all of the damaged valve and some of the heart tissue around it. A replacement valve will be put into the valve opening and then sewn into place.

- After the valve is repaired or replaced, the incision in the heart or aorta will be closed.

- The surgery team will restart your heart. When it is beating successfully, you will be disconnected from the heart-lung machine, and the surgeon will wire your breastbone together and sew up the chest incision.

- You will be taken to the Intensive Care Unit (ICU) where you will be monitored. You will have a breathing tube in your throat, drainage tubes, a bladder catheter to drain your urine, IV lines, and lines connecting you to a heart monitor.

Recovery

Recovery time after valve surgery varies from one person to the next. It is not uncommon for a patient to stand up and take a few steps within 24 hours after surgery. As you begin to recover, you will be disconnected from various tubes and then moved to a cardiac unit until you are ready to go home. Your doctor will talk with you about how long you need to stay in the hospital and what kind of in-hospital rehabilitation you will have.

It is likely to take at least 6 to 8 weeks before you can return to all of your normal activities. For some people, the improvement in blood flow makes them feel so much better that they can actually do more than they could before their surgery. Others will feel weakened by the surgery for several months. You should not push yourself too hard or too quickly.

Follow your doctor's instructions carefully after you return home, and be sure to take the medications prescribed for you on a regular schedule. Most people who have valve replacement surgery take an anticlotting medication afterward to prevent blood clots from forming around the new valve. Dosages will need to be measured and adjusted regularly to make sure they are not too high or too low. For more information on recovering after surgery, see chapter 7.

Heart Transplant

If your heart is damaged beyond repair, in the last stages of cardiomyopathy, or in severe heart failure, you may be a candidate for heart transplantation. Although the success rate for patients who receive a heart transplant is good (more than 80 percent are alive one year later, and more than 70 percent are alive three years later), it is still a surgery of last resort. A transplant will be recommended only if other treatments have not worked and you would die without a new heart.

Currently, there are less than 2,500 heart transplants done every year in the United States. But according to the American Heart Association, 16,000 people under age 55 need a heart transplant each year. There simply aren't enough hearts for everyone who needs a transplant.

If you are selected as a candidate for a heart transplant, you will begin the waiting process for a donor heart. Whether you get a new heart—and how quickly—will depend on your condition and on the availability of a donor heart that matches your tissue and blood type.

Most patients wait for a transplant at home, but it isn't unusual to be hospitalized for some or all of the waiting period. If you wait at home, you may carry a pager so you can be reached immediately when a donor heart becomes available for you. Your doctor will see you frequently during the waiting period to treat your heart failure and to make sure your condition isn't getting any worse. When a heart is available, you will come to the hospital immediately for the transplant.

A medical team will remove the heart from the donor (usually someone who has just died in an accident), pack it in ice, and bring it to your hospital for the surgery. While that medical team is getting the donor heart, you will be prepared for surgery. You will be given general anesthesia and will quickly fall into a deep sleep. The surgeon will open your chest through the breastbone and expose the heart. A heart-lung machine will be connected to your aorta. This machine will supply oxygen to your blood and circulate the blood throughout your body. After the heart-lung machine takes over, the surgeon will remove your heart and put the donor heart in its place.

Since the donor heart is new to your body, there is a risk that your body will reject it. New antirejection drugs have been developed that greatly reduce this risk, but the possibility is always there. You will need to take antirejection drugs for the rest of your life.

If your heart is so diseased that it looks like you have no chance, a heart transplant can offer hope. But it is a very serious surgery, and after the transplant you will need to take special care of your heart and your body. Your failing heart may have caused other parts of your body to weaken because they were not getting enough blood, and a new heart may not be able to reverse that.

LVAD (Left Ventricular Assist Device)

What's an LVAD?

The wait for a donor heart can be very long. During the wait, your heart failure may weaken your whole body, making surgery too risky. A left ventricular assist device (LVAD) could help you stay alive during the wait, and even regain some health.

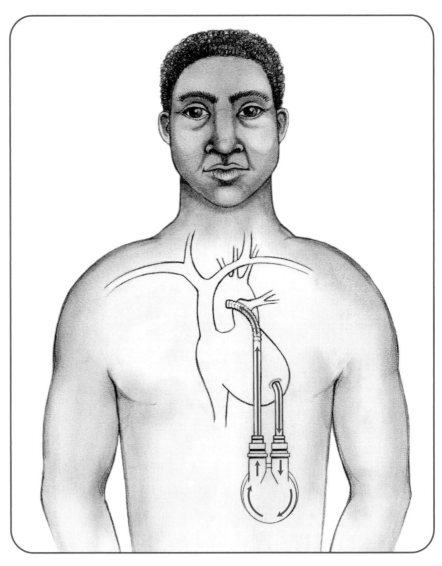

Patients waiting for a heart transplant may have an LVAD implanted. This device will keep blood pumping throughout the body until a donor heart becomes available.

An LVAD is a mechanical device that helps your heart pump blood to the rest of your body. It often is used in patients who are waiting for a heart transplant. Most people with an LVAD are able to wait at home for a transplant.

The LVAD is implanted in the upper part of your abdomen, with one tube going to your left ventricle and another tube going to your aorta. Blood is drawn through the tube in the ventricle into the mechanical pump. It is then sent into the aorta, where it is pumped to the rest of your body. A special driveline connects the pump to its control system, which remains outside your body. The driveline comes out of your abdomen near the waist, on your right side.

In some patients, the LVAD may be a substitute for transplantation. Although it's odd to think of a machine replacing your heart, it may be a solution—either temporary or permanent—for the current shortage of donor hearts.

NEW THERAPIES AND RESEARCH

A great deal of research into new therapies is going on all the time. There are exciting possibilities for new drugs, better ways to do surgery, and nonsurgical alternatives for even very serious heart disease.

Some of these therapies may work well, some may only work for certain people, and some may be dangerous. You should never try a new therapy—not even if it sounds harmless—without talking to your doctor first.

It makes sense to stay informed about new therapies for heart disease. If you find something that sounds interesting, discuss it with your doctor. The therapy may work for you, or it may not be right for your condition.

If you are willing to take part in an experiment, tell your doctor. Sometimes researchers are looking for patients who are willing to test new drugs or other therapies. Although any new therapy carries certain risks, researchers will explain the risks so you can decide if you want to participate.

Gene Therapy

Researchers are trying to alter genes so the heart will one day grow new blood vessels that can bypass narrowed arteries. Although the research is still very new, many scientists are excited about the possibility of patients growing "natural" bypasses.

New Drugs

Several new drugs have been developed to help stop blood clots. Used after angioplasty, these drugs have been shown to reduce the chances of death or serious complications. Some researchers are looking at how to use these new drugs, sometimes called "super aspirin," with clot-dissolving drugs in patients who have just had a heart attack.

Vitamin E

Some interesting new research shows that vitamin E, a part of our daily diet, helps reduce "free radicals," harmful proteins that can damage small blood vessels throughout the body. Some doctors are recommending that their patients take vitamin E tablets every day. Talk to your doctor about whether this might be helpful to you.

LVAD (Left Ventricular Assist Device)

The LVAD is often used in patients waiting for a heart transplant. But researchers have found that in some cases, an LVAD so improves a patient's condition that he or she no longer needs a transplant. Sometimes, damaged heart cells actually recover. In the future, more and more patients may be able to use the LVAD instead of undergoing heart transplantation.

Laser Treatment (Transmyocardial Revascularization, or TMR)

For some patients, heart laser surgery may relieve severe angina. A cardiac surgeon makes an incision in the chest, then uses a high-powered laser to make 20 to 45 small holes in the heart muscle. These small holes seem to stimulate the formation of new blood vessels, improving blood flow and oxygen to the heart. This relieves angina, although the reason why is not yet fully understood.

TMR is done while the heart is beating. It can be used for patients who continue to have severe angina after other treatments have failed. Although still experimental, TMR seems to successfully reduce angina without open heart surgery.

Enhanced External Counterpulsation (EECP)

With enhanced external counterpulsation, external pressure is used to move blood through the body so the heart doesn't have to work as hard.

An inflatable cuff is wrapped around the legs. When the heart is at rest, the cuff is quickly inflated from the calf to the upper thigh. This squeezing helps push more blood into the heart. When the heart begins to contract, the cuff is quickly deflated, reducing the pressure and making it easier for the heart to pump blood out to the body. With EECP, the heart receives more oxygen, and it doesn't have to work as hard.

This treatment is promising because it is noninvasive; it requires no surgery or hospitalization. For some patients, EECP treatments can help the body develop detours around clogged arteries, creating natural bypasses.

CHAPTER SIX

HEART RHYTHMS

At times, you may become aware of the beat, or rhythm, of your heart. Your morning jog, a fender bender, or a heated argument with your boss all might set your heart pounding.

A complex electrical system in the body controls the rhythm of the heart, keeping it at a normal rhythm most of the time, speeding it up when you exert yourself, and slowing it down when you are at rest.

Although an abnormal rhythm can cause problems, today's technology offers a number of devices that can help control heart rhythm and, in many cases, bring it back to normal.

In this chapter you will learn:

How your heart's rhythm is created.

Important abnormal heart rhythms.

The methods used to diagnose an arrhythmia.

How a pacemaker works.

NORMAL RHYTHM

The beat of your heart is started by an electrical charge. This charge normally originates in the sinoatrial (SA) node, a collection of special cells located in the right atrium. The electrical charge, or impulse, travels through the atria, causing them to contract, then continues to the atrioventricular (AV) node, where it is slowed briefly to allow blood to flow into the ventricles. Then the impulse travels rapidly through the ventricles, causing a contraction that pumps blood to the lungs and body. When the heartbeat is finished, the muscle recharges and starts the process over again.

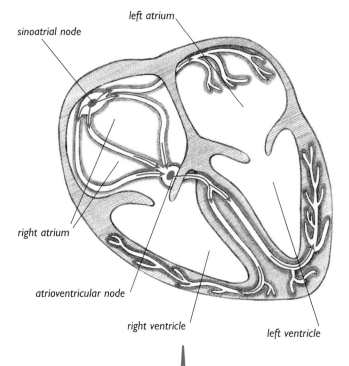

left atrium

sinoatrial node

right atrium

atrioventricular node

right ventricle

left ventricle

A heartbeat, then, is composed of two contractions in your heart: first the atria contract, pushing blood into the ventricles, and then the ventricles contract, pushing blood out into your body.

A normal resting heart rate is between 60 and 100 beats per minute. If you become more active, or if you experience strong emotions (such as fear, excitement, or anxiety), your heart rate will increase. When you sleep, your heart rate will decrease.

ARRHYTHMIA

Arrhythmias are conditions where the heart rate and/or rhythm are abnormal. This can mean your heart is beating too fast, too slow, or irregularly. Arrhythmias can produce a wide variety of symptoms. Some people have arrhythmias without even knowing it. Others feel "skipped" heartbeats, fluttering in their chest, or light-headedness. In worst case scenarios, some arrhythmias can cause people to pass out or even die.

How do I know if I have an arrhythmia?

Bradycardia

A slow heart rate, less than 60 beats per minute, is called bradycardia. It can be fairly harmless. (In fact, some very athletic people have a slow heart rate and it doesn't affect them). But if your heart rate is too slow, it may mean that your body isn't getting enough oxygen.

Tachycardia

A fast heart rate, more than 100 beats per minute, is called tachycardia. There are different kinds of tachycardias, caused by electrical charges originating in different parts of the heart.

Premature Contractions

A premature contraction is an early heartbeat, caused when some part of the heart other than the SA node starts the electrical impulse too soon. You may not feel anything different with this heartbeat, or you may feel as if you have "skipped" a beat. If you

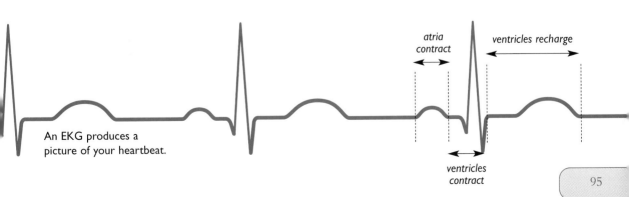

An EKG produces a
picture of your heartbeat.

atria
contract

ventricles recharge

ventricles
contract

don't have heart disease, a premature contraction may not be dangerous. But if you do, premature contractions may be the first stage of another, more serious, arrhythmia.

Supraventricular Tachycardia (SVT)

SVT is a form of tachycardia in which the electrical impulse begins not in the SA node, but in one of the atria or in the AV node. This increases the heart rate, allowing less time for the heart chambers to fill with blood, so less blood is pumped into the heart and body. SVT can last for a few minutes or even a few hours, and is usually quite uncomfortable. You may feel weak or dizzy, or you may have chest discomfort. A fast heart rate along with any of these symptoms requires immediate treatment.

Atrial Fibrillation

Although atrial fibrillation is a fairly common arrhythmia, it can be serious, especially if you have other heart disease. With atrial fibrillation, the atria quiver with many electrical impulses firing 350 to 400 times a minute. Some of these impulses are conducted to the ventricles, resulting in an irregular heart rhythm.

Atrial fibrillation should be treated, because it is linked to heart failure and an increased risk of stroke (when a blood clot blocks an artery to the brain). Symptoms of atrial fibrillation can include heart palpitations, dizziness, and chest pain.

Ventricular Fibrillation

Ventricular fibrillation is a life-threatening emergency. It happens when the ventricles suddenly beat in a fast and irregular way. Blood is not being pumped from the heart, and the heart will stop without immediate treatment. With immediate cardiopulmonary resuscitation (CPR) and an electrical shock to the chest, the heart may be restarted to a normal rhythm.

DIAGNOSING ARRHYTHMIAS

Arrhythmias usually are diagnosed with a simple electrocardiogram or echocardiogram (described in chapter 4.) To check for an arrhythmia, your doctor may use a Holter monitor, Event monitor, tilt table, or electrophysiology study.

Noninvasive Tests

Holter and Event Monitors

Holter and Event monitors are used to get an electrocardiogram over time as you go about your normal activities. With a Holter monitor, you wear a small device that keeps track of your heart rate for 24 hours or more. With an Event monitor, which may be kept for weeks at a time, you push a button whenever you feel symptoms of an irregular heartbeat. In both cases, your doctor will interpret your results.

Tilt Table

Using a tilt table, your doctor may do an electrocardiogram while you are tilted in different positions. You start out lying flat on the table, and as the angle of the table changes, your doctor takes heart rate and blood pressure readings to see how your heart responds.

Invasive Tests

Electrophysiology Study

An electrophysiology (EP) study may be done to better evaluate what appears to be a serious abnormal heart rhythm. An EP study is an internal electrocardiogram using electrodes that have been placed in the heart itself. This test is an integral part of catheter ablation, discussed later in this section.

In this procedure, a doctor threads catheters (thin tubes) through a vein until they are inserted in the heart. The catheters have electrodes on their tips, which can read the electrical impulses created in the heart.

How risky is
an EP study?

Although any procedure that involves inserting something into the heart carries risks, an EP study is very safe. Your healthcare team has the experience and equipment to treat any complications that may arise. Many people have uncomfortable symptoms after an EP study, like a rapid heartbeat or a dizzy feeling, but these do not last long.

TREATING ARRHYTHMIAS

Antiarrhythmic Drugs

If you have an arrhythmia, there are a number of medications that can help regulate your heart rate. It is important to take antiarrhythmic medication exactly as instructed. You should take the medication at the times your doctor has prescribed and only in the dosage prescribed.

It is very important for your doctor to know of any other medications you are taking—even over-the-counter drugs or herbal remedies—because these may affect the way antiarrhythmics work in your body.

Some antiarrhythmics that may be prescribed for you include:

- **Sotalol (Betapace),** which is used for a heart rate that is too fast. Its side effects can include fatigue, shortness of breath, dizziness, impotence, and an increased heart rate. If you have diabetes, be aware that sotalol can hide some symptoms of low blood sugar.

- **Propafenone (Rythmol),** which is used for an irregular heartbeat or to prevent the reoccurrence of an arrhythmia. If you are taking other heart medications, you need to have your blood levels checked regularly. Possible side effects include an irregular heart rate, slow heart rate, shortness of breath, nausea, vomiting, a metallic taste, constipation, dizziness, fatigue, chest pain, headache, and blurred vision.

- **Procainamide (Pronestyl-SR or Procanbid),** which is used to help an irregular heart rate become more regular and to slow a heart that is beating too quickly. Possible side effects include nausea, dizziness, diarrhea, loss of appetite, and weakness. You should call your doctor if you have chills, fever, joint pain, itching, skin rash, or difficulty breathing.

- **Flecainide (Tambocor),** which can help an irregular heartbeat become more regular. Possible side effects include dizziness, blurred vision, constipation, nausea, or headache. You should call your doctor if you experience fever, chest pain, shortness of breath, trembling, swelling of your feet or legs, or yellowing of your eyes or skin.

- **Amiodarone (Cordarone),** which is used for irregular heartbeats. This medication will make your skin more sensitive to sun. Avoid direct sunlight, or use a special zinc- or titanium-oxide sunscreen if you must be in the sun. Possible side effects include sunburn (even in winter), thyroid disorders, yellowing of the eyes or skin, lung problems, trembling, constipation, difficulty with balance, fever, headache, vomiting, nausea, a fast or irregular heartbeat, blurry vision, and a temporary drop in blood pressure.

Cardioversion

For a rapid or irregular heart rhythm that isn't helped by medication, cardioversion may be required. This is an electric shock that changes your heart rhythm and allows your heart to resume a normal rate.

Cardioversion is done while you are sedated. Paddles or electrode pads are placed on your chest and back, and an electric shock is delivered to change the rhythm of your heart. There is no pain during the shock, but your chest may feel sore afterward.

Implantable Devices

In the past couple of decades, implantable devices have been developed to keep your heart beating in a normal rhythm. Pacemakers can be used to speed up a heart that is beating too slowly, and defibrillators may be used to interrupt a heart rhythm that is too fast.

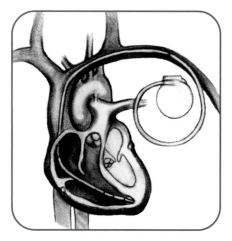

A single-chamber pacemaker has one lead that generally goes into the right ventricle.

Pacemaker

A cardiac pacemaker is a device that sends electrical impulses to keep your heart rate within a normal range. It is most often used in cases of bradycardia (a slow heart rate). Pacemakers have been refined over the years, and today's versions are very reliable and very small, about the size of a silver dollar.

The pacemaker itself is a small metal case containing a battery, electric circuits, and a computer-like sensor that lets the pacemaker know when to send an electric impulse. One or two leads (thin wires) are threaded through a vein, placed inside your heart, and then attached to the pacemaker. At the tip of each lead is an electrode that senses the heart's activity and sends out electric impulses when they are needed.

A *single-chamber pacemaker* has one lead that usually goes into the right ventricle. A *dual-chamber pacemaker* has two leads; one is placed in the right atrium, the other in the right ventricle.

A *rate-responsive pacemaker* recognizes that your heart rate should vary according to your level of activity. If you are walking briskly, for example, your heart needs to beat at a faster pace than if you are quietly reading a book.

If your doctor thinks a pacemaker will help with your heart rhythm, you will be scheduled for surgery. Most likely your doctor will implant the pacemaker near your collarbone. For certain patients, the doctor may implant the pacemaker in the lower abdomen.

Your doctor can adjust your pacemaker through an external control system; you will not need an operation for this. However, when the battery becomes low, you will need to have the whole pacemaker replaced, because the battery is sealed inside the pacemaker. Your doctor will monitor the pacemaker at regular visits and prepare to replace it before the battery wears out, generally within 8 to 10 years.

Most people can have a normal life with a pacemaker—some even take part in fairly strenuous sports. Talk to your doctor about what kind of activities you can do and what you may need to avoid.

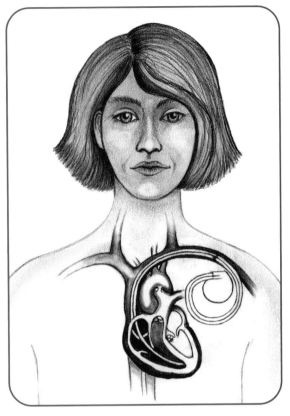

A dual-chamber pacemaker has two leads—one embedded in the right atrium, the other in the right ventricle.

You will be given a pacemaker-patient identification card. Keep this with you at all times. If you need emergency medical attention, those who are treating you should know that you have a pacemaker.

Strong electromagnetic fields (interference from electrical equipment and devices) can affect your pacemaker. When you move away from the interference, your pacemaker will go back to its normal operation.

Is my pacemaker safe around a microwave? Most equipment in your home or workplace will not cause a problem for your pacemaker—not even your microwave oven. You should, however, be careful around:

- Electric arc welding equipment.

- The ignition system of your car or other internal combustion engine.

- Cellular phones. (The research is mixed, but there are signs that cellular phones may interfere with your pacemaker. If you must use a cellular phone, you might avoid problems by keeping it at least 6 inches from where the pacemaker is implanted, and by using the ear opposite the side of your pacemaker.)

Your car's seatbelt may press against your pacemaker when you put it on. This is not dangerous to you or harmful to the pacemaker, but it may feel uncomfortable for the first weeks after the pacemaker is implanted. You may want to place a towel or piece of foam between the belt and the pacemaker. DO NOT stop using your seatbelt.

Before undergoing medical or dental work, tell your doctor, dentist, or technician that you have a pacemaker. Most procedures will not cause problems, but healthcare professionals may need to take precautions.

Defibrillator
An implantable cardiac defibrillator (ICD) is a small device—about the size of a pager—that can break up impulses that are too fast or inconsistent. Such impulses, or fibrillations, make your heart rhythm go out of control, and you may lose consciousness if they aren't interrupted.

In an emergency setting, an external defibrillator is used to send a shock that will stop fibrillation. (You may have seen this on television or in the movies.) The ICD essentially provides the same function, except that it can stop fibrillation from within your chest.

The ICD can be a lifesaver—literally—for people with serious cardiac arrhythmias. Having an ICD will not greatly limit your everyday activities; in fact, it will probably increase your ability to live your life normally.

The ICD can be used in several ways:

- It can be programmed to give small shocks, or pacing signals, if it detects a fast rhythm. This is called *antitachycardia pacing*. The series of small shocks is intended to restore normal rhythm to your heart. You probably won't feel the shocks, but if you do, you won't find them painful.

    Will I feel the shocks coming from my ICD?

- It can be programmed to give stronger shocks if pacing does not stop the rapid beating of your heart. This is called *cardioversion*. This kind of shock will probably feel uncomfortable, as if you've just been thumped on the chest.

- It can be programmed to give a high-energy shock that will interrupt fibrillation and give the heart a chance to go back to a normal rhythm. If you are conscious when you get a defibrillating shock—and you may have lost consciousness with the fibrillation—you will feel the shock like a strong blow or kick to your chest. It goes away quickly, however.

The ICD, which is made of titanium, is implanted under the skin or muscles in your upper chest or your abdomen. The main part of the ICD looks like a shiny box about the size of a 9-volt battery. Inside is a tiny computer and a battery to supply power. The "battery pack" will have one or more leads (thin wires) that are threaded through a vein into your heart.

Using an external control system, the doctor can program—and reprogram—the computer in your ICD. The doctor can also access your heart-rhythm information, which is stored inside the ICD.

You will be given an ICD-patient identification card. Keep this with you at all times. If you need emergency medical attention, those who are treating you should know that you have an ICD.

If your ICD delivers a shock to your heart, as it's supposed to during a rapid or irregular heart pattern, you may need to sit or lie down for a while. Ask your doctor if you should call each time you feel a shock from your ICD. Tell your family, friends, and coworkers how they can help you after you receive a shock.

Some people may not be able to drive because of their arrhythmia and the shocks delivered by the ICD.

You must avoid strong electromagnetic fields. These can prevent the ICD from delivering treatment when needed, or they can cause it to give a shock when it shouldn't. The ICD should work normally as soon as you move away from the electromagnetic field. You might experience problems with the following:

- Industrial equipment.

- Arc and resistance welders.

- Large magnets.

- Antennas used for CB, ham radio, or other transmitters.

- Large television or radio transmitting towers.

- Power lines carrying more than 100,000 volts. (Stay at least 25 feet away.)

- Some medical procedures, such as radiation therapy or magnetic resonance imaging.

- Hand-held screening wands at airports. (You can safely walk through the security screen archway, but a hand-held wand has a magnet in it.)

- Cellular phones. (The research is mixed, but there are signs that cellular phones can interfere with an ICD. If you must use a cellular phone, you might avoid problems by keeping the phone at least 6 inches from where the ICD is implanted, and by using the ear on the opposite side of your ICD.)

Before having any medical or dental work done, you need to tell your doctor, dentist, or technician that you have an ICD. Most medical and dental work will not cause problems, but healthcare professionals may need to take safety measures if you have an ICD.

Catheter Ablation

Some people experience a fast heart rate along with lightheadedness, faintness, shortness of breath, chest pain, or chest pressure. This condition may be treated by ablating (burning out) certain cells in the heart in order to stop them from conducting too many impulses.

If your doctor determines that this procedure would help, you will be scheduled for an electrophysiology study (described earlier in this section) and a catheter ablation. During the electrophysiology study, catheters will be inserted into a vein or artery in your neck or groin and then threaded carefully toward your heart. Once the doctor has located the area of your heart that is causing the problem, a special catheter will be inserted into that site. Radio frequency waves are sent through the catheter to "burn out" a small area of heart tissue. This is called *catheter ablation*.

Catheter ablation is not painful and is likely to be done without anesthetic, although you may be given a sedative to keep you calm. Because the procedure varies from one patient to another, your healthcare providers will give you specific information about your procedure. Catheter ablation generally takes from 2 to 6 hours.

Catheter ablation usually brings very good results. You may still feel an occasional "skipped" heartbeat for a few months, but in most cases, ablation eliminates the problem.

If you have atrial fibrillation and your heart rate cannot be controlled through medication, ablation may be used to block the conduction of your heart's electrical impulses. For this reason, you may need a pacemaker to ensure a normal heart rate. The pacemaker will likely be implanted at the time of your ablation.

CHAPTER SEVEN

JOURNEY TO BETTER HEALTH

Having a heart problem, whether it's an occasional irregular rhythm or a heart attack, almost always means making some changes in your life. If you haven't been leading a "heart healthy" life already, you need to start now.

You may groan at the idea of changing your diet or getting out to exercise, but lifestyle changes that are good for your heart are good for the rest of you, too. Eating a healthy, balanced diet, getting regular exercise, giving up smoking, and moderating your use of alcohol can help you not only live longer, but live better.

In this chapter you will learn:

What a "heart healthy" diet is.

How to fit regular exercise into your life.

The importance of taking your medications.

When to call your doctor.

AFTER A CARDIAC OPERATION

If you have had a coronary bypass, valve replacement, or any other major cardiac surgery, you will need to take special care when you get home from the hospital. During the first week at home, you will have to pay particular attention to how your surgical wound is healing.

General Care

Is it okay to shower before my surgical wound has healed?

- You should take a shower—not a bath—every day, but use only antibacterial soap like Dial, Safeguard, or Zest. Remove all your dressings before you shower. Don't put any lotion, powder, ointment, oil, or medication on your incisions unless your surgeon says it's okay.

- Inspect your incisions every day. Call your surgeon if you see increased redness, tenderness, swelling, warmth, drainage, or separation. Keep your incisions out of direct sunlight for at least 8 weeks, and use sunscreen on them after that.

- Take your temperature daily and record it on the log on the following page. You may wish to copy the log and keep the pages in a notebook to bring to your doctor appointments.

- Weigh yourself before breakfast, after you have used the bathroom for the first time in the morning. Use the log on the next page to record your daily weight. If you gain 2 to 3 pounds overnight, or 3 to 5 pounds during the week, call your doctor.

- Wear elastic stockings during the day, if your doctor has ordered them. Do not wear them at night and do not put them on by yourself.

Daily Weight and Temperature Log

DATE	TEMPERATURE	WEIGHT

Living Well with Heart Disease © 2000 Fairview Press

Medications

- Take pain pills as prescribed by your doctor.

- Get your doctor's approval before taking any over-the-counter medications, herbs, or vitamins.

- You can use a stool softener for 3 to 4 weeks to relieve constipation. Your doctor may recommend one. Do not take a laxative without your doctor's permission.

Diet

- Avoid very salty foods, which may cause you to retain fluids.

Activity

- You may lie on your side if it feels comfortable, and if there is no "click" in your breastbone.

- Do the exercises given to you by your cardiac rehabilitation specialist. Avoid lifting, pushing, or pulling anything that weighs more than 5 to 10 pounds.

- Be sure to rest between activities.

- Keep your legs and feet elevated if you sit for more than 10 to 15 minutes. Use a footstool when sitting on a chair or couch.

- Do not drive a vehicle for at least 4 weeks. You must have your doctor's permission before you begin driving again.

Incentive Spirometer

Because of the incision through your breastbone, you may find it somewhat uncomfortable to breathe deeply. As you recover from your surgery, it is important that you learn to breathe normally again.

The incentive spirometer helps you get back to your normal breathing. You will be asked to use the incentive spirometer as soon as you are able to breathe through your mouth in the hospital. The spirometer will be sent home with you, and you will be asked to use it several times each day for the first couple of weeks.

The incentive spirometer has a piston that rises as you inhale through a tube. You can see how much air you are taking in by the height of the piston at the end of each breath.

Here's how to use the incentive spirometer:

How do I use an incentive spirometer?

- Put the mouthpiece of the incentive spirometer in your mouth.

- Inhale slowly and watch the piston rise. Keep inhaling and try to move the piston to the level your doctor or therapist has prescribed. (The top of the piston determines the level you are at.)

- When you have taken in all the air you can, remove the mouthpiece and hold your breath for as long as your doctor or therapist recommends, then exhale normally.

- Let the piston sink back to the bottom of the chamber while you rest.

- Repeat 9 more times, or as recommended.

At home you should use the incentive spirometer at least 3 times each day, for 10 breaths each time. After each session, take a deep breath and then cough as deeply as you can to clear any secretions in your airway. When you cough, support your chest incision with your hand.

When to Call Your Cardiac Care Provider

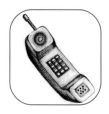

- If you have a temperature of more than 100°F for more than 24 hours.

- If you have a heart rate that is too slow, too fast, or that seems to skip a beat.

- If you are short of breath, even when you rest.

- If you gain over 3 pounds in a day or 5 pounds in a week.

- If you have continued dizziness.

- If you feel chest or shoulder pain that is worse when you breathe deeply or cough.

- If you have swelling, oozing, or other signs of infection around the incision.

- If you suddenly bruise or bleed easily, for no apparent reason.

- If you have blood in your bowel movements, which makes them look dark or tarry, or if your urine is bloody.

- If you have frequent or very bad headaches.

- If you feel chills or shaking.

- If you notice a new or increased shifting, clicking, or popping in your breastbone.

- If your pain medication doesn't ease the pain in your incision or chest area.

- If you suddenly have less energy and endurance.

MEDICATIONS

Medications are important for treating heart disease. Although any drug should be taken as prescribed by your doctor, when it comes to your heart and circulatory system, it's particularly important that you take your medications *exactly* as directed.

You'll find descriptions of common heart medications in chapter 4, with general instructions for their use. Your doctor may prescribe some of these medications, or you may be given a drug that is not on that list. In any case, you should follow your doctor's instructions.

Your doctor may give you a schedule for keeping track of your medications, or you may use the chart on page 68. Carry this with you at all times. Record the name of the drug, the dosage, the time you take it, and any reactions or comments you may have. Bring the schedule to every doctor's visit, so he or she can see that you are taking your medications and determine whether adjustments need to be made.

- **Take each medication exactly as directed.** Don't take two doses at once if you've missed a dose (unless your doctor says it's okay), and don't skip a dose because you're feeling better. Follow the directions given to you by the pharmacist, such as whether to take the medication with food or on an empty stomach, and whether to avoid alcohol.

  What if I miss a dose?

- **Be sure to store drugs as directed.** Some medications are particularly sensitive to heat or humidity.

- **Never share your medication with other people,** even if they have symptoms similar to yours.

- **Make sure every doctor you go to knows which medications you are taking.** If you see a family care physician for something unrelated to your heart disease, it's important that he or she knows what heart medications you are taking.

- **Get all of your prescriptions filled at one place,** so the pharmacy will have a complete record of the medications you are taking. If there's a chance of a dangerous drug interaction, the pharmacist may spot it.

- **Learn as much as you can about each of your medications.** Know their names, their dosages, your reasons for taking them, and possible side effects.

CARDIAC REHABILITATION

Cardiac rehabilitation services are for people who are recovering from a heart attack, bypass surgery, or another heart-related event. These services help you return to your daily life so you are able to work and live at the highest level of physical, psychological, and social functioning that you can.

A heart condition is not something you can just "get past." It requires you to make some changes in your life. You can get started on those changes while you are in the hospital, but most people need help and encouragement after they've gone home.

Inpatient Rehabilitation

This begins in the hospital after a heart attack, heart surgery, or other heart-related incident. The goal of inpatient rehabilitation is to reverse the side effects of bedrest. It includes activities like walking in the hall, walking on a treadmill, or riding a stationary bike.

During inpatient rehabilitation you will learn more about your diagnosis, your risk factors, and how your body responds to exercise, all while being monitored carefully by staff who are experts in rehabilitation.

Outpatient Rehabilitation

Outpatient rehabilitation occurs after you leave the hospital. It includes education, exercise, counseling, and behavioral changes. The goals of outpatient rehabilitation are:

- To improve cardiovascular fitness, endurance, muscle strength, and flexibility.

- To help you develop a healthier lifestyle that includes good nutrition and regular exercise.

- To modify lifestyle choices that increase your risk of heart disease, such as smoking.

- To provide emotional support while you go back to your daily activities.

Outpatient rehabilitation is often done in a small group setting, although you will have an individual care plan to meet your specific needs.

The First Few Weeks

During your first few weeks home from the hospital, you may tire easily. Let your body guide you. When you feel tired, you need to take a rest. Follow the "One hour and 10 minute rule": If you are active for an hour, then sit and take a 10-minute rest. If you have been resting for an hour, then get up and walk around for 10 minutes. A typical day at home should include:

- Light to moderate activities, like simple meal preparation, dressing, washing, a short trip to the store, or a visit with a friend.

- Exercise.

- Rest and relaxation.

When you're planning your day, try to follow these guidelines:

- **Avoid rushing.** Take it easy. A moderate pace is best.

- **Plan ahead.** Allow enough time for each activity.

- **Rest often to avoid getting overtired.**

- **Don't force yourself to finish an activity if you are feeling tired.** Stop and go back to it later.

- **Wait 30 to 60 minutes after eating before you exercise.** The bigger the meal, the longer you should wait.

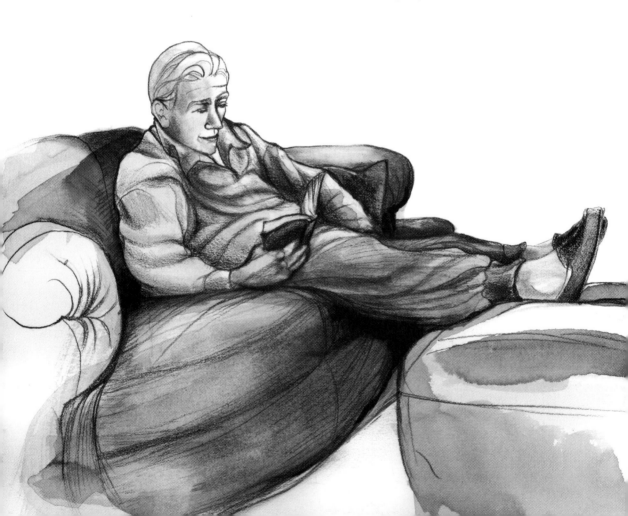

- **Do not participate in strenuous activities** such as lifting weights, moving furniture, shoveling snow, or doing heavy yard work.

- **Don't work or exercise outdoors in very hot or very cold temperatures.** Either extreme will force your body to work too hard. In warm weather, follow the "160 rule": If the outdoor temperature plus the humidity equal 160, you should stay indoors in an air-conditioned place. (For example, if the temperature is 90°F and the humidity is 70 percent, the two numbers add up to 160; therefore, you should avoid outdoor activities.)

- **Remember to breathe.** Yes, it sounds silly, but pay attention to see if you hold your breath as you work or exercise. If you do, try singing or talking to yourself during physical activity to make sure you are breathing in and out.

Work Simplification

When you are recovering from heart surgery, you need to save your energy and take extra care not to get overtired, at least for a while. If you have a damaged heart, you may need to change the way you do things.

"Work simplification" is a way of looking at activities around your home or at your workplace and figuring out ways to reduce the amount of energy and movement you need to expend.

- **Planning is essential.** Organize your day so you know what you can get done when. Be sure to schedule time for rest.

- **Get rid of activities that aren't really necessary.** Maybe the dirty windows can wait. Maybe you can make one trip to the copy machine instead of three.

- **Alternate work periods and rest periods throughout the day.** Don't assume you'll work hard all day and then rest.

- **Ask for help when you need it from family, friends, and coworkers.** Let them help organize your tasks, too. They may have ideas about how to simplify or eliminate activities.

- **Pay attention to your posture.** Good posture helps you save energy and feel less tired.

- **Work at a moderate pace.** This is easier than rushing through your work, then finding yourself exhausted. In the long run, it takes about the same amount of time.

Maintenance

Once you're back to "normal," you may need—or want—additional support to help you stick with a healthy diet, regular exercise, and other lifestyle changes.

Community-based cardiac programs often hold group seminars on exercise and nutrition, which are led by cardiac rehabilitation experts. Home programs, tailored to your special needs, also may be available in your area.

DIET

Almost anyone can benefit from a low-fat, low-salt, high-fiber diet. But if you have a heart problem, it is very important for you to eat healthfully. A low-fat, low-cholesterol diet can help lower your overall cholesterol and give your heart a chance.

The American Heart Association recommends its Step II Diet for people with heart disease. This diet is low in saturated fat and cholesterol.

Is Your Diet Heart Healthy?

Use the chart on the following page to determine if your diet is heart healthy—and to see where you can make improvements. For each food group, place a checkmark next to the selection that best represents your eating habits. Then, count the number of checkmarks you made in each column. If the majority are in:

Level 1: Take a good look at your eating habits. You are probably eating too many foods that are high in fat, cholesterol, calories, and salt. See if you can advance to Level 2 by making small changes in each group.

Level 2: Good job. You are moving in the right direction. At this level you are eating many good foods that are lower in fat, cholesterol, calories, and salt. To improve your eating habits even more, work toward Level 3.

Level 3: You have reached the American Heart Association Step II Diet. Keep up the good work and use your creativity to help family and friends stay interested in healthier eating. If you want a diet even lower in fat and cholesterol, keep on working toward Level 4 (but be sure to speak to a dietitian first).

Level 4: You have reached a vegetarian diet that is high in fiber, low in sodium and cholesterol, and no more than 10 percent fat. Be sure to speak with a dietitian to make sure you're getting adequate nutrition with this diet.

The Basics of Eating Healthy

The food pyramid, developed by the USDA, is a basic tool for developing a healthy diet. You can tell by looking at the food pyramid that breads, pasta, rice, fruits, and vegetables should be the main part of your diet.

Four Levels of Diet

Food Group	Level 1	Level 2	Level 3	Level 4
Fresh/frozen fruits and vegetables	___ 0–1 servings a day	___ 2–3 servings a day	___ 5 or more servings a day	___ 5 or more servings a day
Canned soups or vegetables	___ 4 or more times a week	___ 1–3 times a week	___ Less than 2 g fat, 600 mg sodium per serving	___ Less than 2 g fat, 600 mg sodium per serving
Bread, cereal, rice, whole grains, pasta	___ Once a day or less	___ 2–3 servings a day	___ 6 or more servings a day	___ 6 or more servings a day
Dried beans and peas, tofu	___ Rarely or never	___ Once a week	___ 2 or more times a week	___ Daily
Milk	___ 2% or whole	___ 1%	___ Skim	___ Skim
Cheese	___ Mainly high-fat cheese (Swiss, Colby, cheddar, American)	___ Mainly low-fat cheese	___ Only nonfat or low-fat cheese, or eat cheese rarely	___ Only nonfat cheese, or eat cheese rarely
Poultry (no skin, not fried), fish (not fried)	___ Once a week or less	___ 1–2 servings a week	___ 2 or more 3-oz servings a week	___ Avoid
Red meat	___ Mainly high-fat meats (sausage, hamburger, lunch meats, ham, hot dogs)	___ Mainly lean meats (85% lean ground or round steak)	___ Only lean meats (beef, chuck roast, flank, pork loin roast)	___ Avoid
Eggs	___ 5 or more egg yolks a week	___ 3–4 egg yolks a week	___ 3 or fewer egg yolks a week	___ Avoid egg yolks
Cooking oils and fats	___ Use butter, shortening, or lard for cooking and eating	___ Use margarine or vegetable oil for cooking and eating	___ Only margarine or liquid vegetable oils. No more than 6–8 tsp a day	___ Up to 3 tsps a day nonfat margarine or cooking oil (safflower, canola)
Baked goods and desserts	___ Frequent commercial baked goods and desserts	___ Only low-fat baked goods and desserts	___ Avoid, or eat foods with negligible fat	___ Avoid, or eat only nonfat baked goods and desserts

Living Well with Heart Disease © 2000 Fairview Press

For many of us, this is a pretty big change. We are used to building our meals around meat, not around vegetables. Improving our diet means making a conscious decision to:

How can I improve my diet?

- Use more fresh or frozen fruits and vegetables.

- Use more foods made from whole grains.

- Read food labels. Today's food labels can help you keep track of fat, sodium, and cholesterol so you can eat a healthy diet.

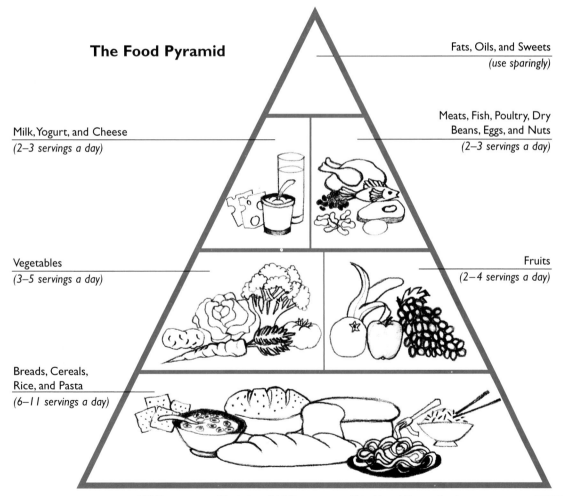

The Food Pyramid

Fats, Oils, and Sweets
(use sparingly)

Milk, Yogurt, and Cheese
(2–3 servings a day)

Meats, Fish, Poultry, Dry Beans, Eggs, and Nuts
(2–3 servings a day)

Vegetables
(3–5 servings a day)

Fruits
(2–4 servings a day)

Breads, Cereals, Rice, and Pasta
(6–11 servings a day)

U.S. Department of Agriculture/U.S. Department of Health and Human Services

Low Fat

You can't eliminate fat from your diet, and you shouldn't. Fat gives you energy and provides your body with the materials it needs to build cell walls, process vitamins, and more.

Is all fat bad?

There are "bad fats" (saturated fats) and "good fats" (unsaturated fats). *Saturated fats* are found in meats, whole milk dairy products, and some oils. *Unsaturated fats* can be found in vegetable oils, fish, and nuts.

There are two kinds of unsaturated fats: *polyunsaturated fats,* in such foods as soybean oil, corn oil, and safflower oil; and *monounsaturated fats,* in such foods as olives, avocados, and nuts.

Although unsaturated fats are better for your heart than saturated fats, any kind of fat can raise your cholesterol level.

Most Americans eat too much fat. The American Heart Association and the National Cholesterol Education Program recommend that no more than 30 percent of your total daily calories come from fat. For most people, a low-fat diet means:

How much fat should I eat?

- If you are a man, no more than 50 to 60 grams of fat each day.

- If you are a woman, no more than 40 to 50 grams of fat each day.

Nutrition labels on food products, such as the one on the following page, will tell you how many calories are in a typical serving, and how many of those calories come from fat. After eating a heart healthy diet for a while, you will have a pretty good sense of how to cut back on fat. But at first you may need to write down the total calories you eat every day—as well as the calories from fat—in order to make sure you're limiting the amount of fat in your diet.

Nutrition Facts

Serving Size 1 cup (228g)
Servings Per Container 2

Amount Per Serving

Calories 90	Calories from Fat 30

	% Daily Value★
Total Fat 3g	**5%**
Saturated Fat 0g	**0%**
Cholesterol 0mg	**0%**
Sodium 300mg	**13%**
Total Carbohydrate 13g	**4%**
Dietary Fiber 3g	**12%**
Sugars 3g	
Protein 3g	

Vitamin A 80%	•	Vitamin C 60%
Calcium 4%	•	Iron 4%

★ Percent Daily Values are based on a 2,000
calorie diet. Your daily values may be higher
or lower depending on your calorie needs.

	Calories	2,000	2,500
Total Fat	Less than	65g	80g
Sat Fat	Less than	20g	25g
Cholesterol	Less than	300mg	300mg
Sodium	Less than	2,400mg	2,400mg
Total Carbohydrate		300g	375g
Dietary Fiber		25g	30g

Calories per gram
Fat 9 • Carbohydrate 4 • Protein 4

When reading food labels, compare the serving size to the amount you are eating. You will need to adjust the numbers if you eat more or less than the serving size listed on the label.

You can reduce the amount of fat in your diet and still have interesting, tasty meals:

- Eat no more than 6 ounces a day of fish, poultry, or lean meat, and try to eat meatless meals throughout the week.

- Always trim fat from meat, and take the skin off chicken or poultry (much of the fat is in the skin).

- Roast, bake, broil, boil, or steam foods instead of frying them.

- Eat no more than 3 egg yolks a week.

- Look for low-fat or nonfat dairy products. Switch to skim or 1 percent milk.

- Limit foods made with coconut, palm, or palm kernel oils.

- Choose low-fat, whole-grain breads, cereals, and crackers.

- Eat at least 5 servings of fruits and vegetables every day.

- Limit your use of fats and oils in cooking and in salad dressings. Use no more than 3 to 4 teaspoons of added fat each day.

Food manufacturers have made it easier to watch the fat in your diet and to choose low-fat options. You can avoid egg yolks and still have scrambled eggs, for example, by picking up an egg substitute from the dairy section in your grocery store.

Dozens of cookbooks offer low-fat, delicious, easy-to-make recipes—simply browse your nearest bookstore, or see the list at the back of this book.

Low Sodium

When we think of sodium, we usually think of table salt. That's natural, since table salt is 40 percent sodium. But sodium is also found in many foods. Some foods, like tomatoes, naturally contain sodium. Processed foods, like hot dogs and frozen waffles, are likely to have sodium added as a preservative.

The American Heart Association Step II Diet recommends no more than 2,400 milligrams of sodium per day. A teaspoon of salt contains 2,300 milligrams of sodium. To limit the amount of sodium in your diet:

- Stop using the salt shaker.

- Cut back on high-sodium flavorings like MSG and soy sauce.

- Avoid foods that contain baking soda or baking powder.

- Use sodium-free spices and seasonings. A number of manufacturers now make spice mixes that add taste to your food without adding sodium. Or try some "good old-fashioned" seasonings such as lemon, garlic, and onion.

- Don't use a salt substitute without talking to your doctor first. Salt substitutes contain potassium, which may be a problem with some medications.

  Should I use a salt substitute?

- Stock up on fresh fruits and vegetables.

- Avoid canned vegetables.

- Cut back on processed foods. Although they are convenient, most are high in sodium.

- Read food labels carefully and keep track of the amount of sodium you eat every day.

High Fiber

A high-fiber diet (20 to 35 grams of fiber per day) may help protect against heart disease—and other diseases as well. If you eat a healthy diet based on the Food Pyramid, you will have plenty of fiber. Cereals, bran, and whole-wheat products are high in fiber. So are most fruits and vegetables.

Fiber tends to make you feel full, and most fiber-rich foods have little or no fat. If you need to lose weight as part of your treatment for heart problems, eating fiber can help you lose weight without feeling deprived.

If you have had a low-fiber diet until now, adding a lot of fiber at once can cause gas, bloating, or diarrhea. These are temporary problems, but you might avoid them by gradually switching to high-fiber foods.

EXERCISE

It's no surprise that exercise is good for you. Whether you work out every day at the health club, or it's a major effort just to walk from the couch to the refrigerator, you know you should have regular exercise in your life.

You may hesitate at the thought of exercising when you have heart disease or when you're recovering from heart surgery, but exercise is an important step on the road back to health.

When can I start exercising again?

Before starting any new exercise program, you need to talk with your doctor about your condition and any limitations you may have. Your doctor may refer you to cardiac rehabilitation services.

Walking

One of the best exercises is something you can do at no cost, without fancy equipment, almost anytime and anywhere: walking.

Walking is a form of aerobic exercise. It conditions the heart and lungs, increasing the oxygen available to the body and helping the heart use that oxygen better. Regular aerobic exercise helps the heart pump without having to work too hard. This means that the heart can beat fewer times per minute, but still get the same amount of blood and oxygen to the body. Many premier athletes have relatively low heart rates because their bodies have become so accustomed to exercise that their hearts are now extremely efficient.

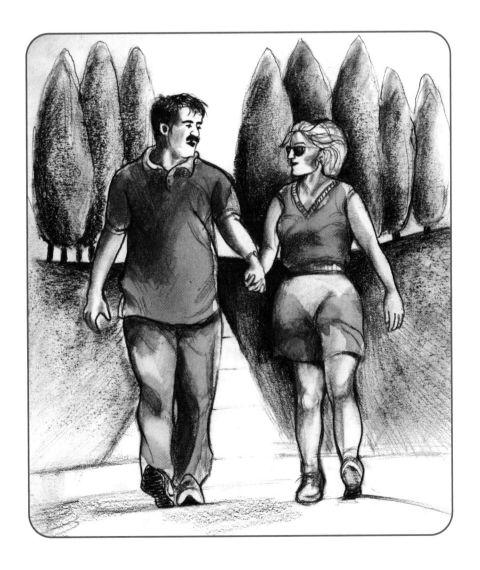

You can walk near your home, or you can walk at a gym or health club. And many shopping centers open early so "mall walkers" can walk safely out of the weather.

You don't need any training to walk, and although you should wear supportive shoes and comfortable clothing, you don't need any special equipment, either.

How can I get in the habit of exercising?

- **Do not start a walking program until your doctor tells you to.** Most people are able to begin a slow program while in the hospital. Your rehabilitation specialist will provide a written program to guide your progress at home.

- **Choose a specific time of day to walk, and stick to it.** Try for the time you have the most energy. If you are a morning person, you may want to walk right after you wake up, as a healthy start to the day. If mornings are a bit sluggish for you, try walking in the midafternoon or sometime before dinner.

- **Find a place, or several places, where you can walk regularly no matter what the weather.**

- **Try to walk in moderate temperatures (indoors or outdoors).** If you must be out in cold weather (below 30°F), use a scarf or face mask. Avoid extreme heat or extreme cold.

- **Consider walking with a partner.** If you think you will be tempted to "skip" walking days, try to find a walking partner who walks at about the same pace you do. Of course, some people prefer solitude while walking—it's a good time to think and reflect—so do what's most satisfying for you.

- **Walk before meals or at least one hour after meals.**

- **If you take nitroglycerin, always bring it along on your walks.**

If walking isn't a realistic or comfortable option, your rehabilitation specialist will help you identify the type of exercise that is best for you.

Toning Exercises

Simple toning exercises can help you stay flexible and healthy. After surgery, these exercises are particularly important for regaining muscle tone and increasing circulation.

Your doctor will tell you when it's okay to start toning exercises. Usually this will be the day after you get home from the hospital, but you may be started on an exercise program sooner. Your rehabilitation specialist will show you how to do the exercises and will give you written directions and diagrams. Stop exercising if you notice:

Is it normal to feel dizzy during exercise?

- Any chest pain, or pain that radiates to your teeth, jaw, ear, or arm. (If you have pain or pressure that doesn't get better with rest, take your nitroglycerin tablets. If there's no relief within 15 minutes of taking the nitroglycerin, call 911 immediately.)

- Lightheadedness, dizziness, or fainting spells during or after exercise.

- Irregular heartbeats or palpitations.

- Exhaustion or extreme fatigue.

- Weight gain of 3 to 5 pounds in three days or less.

- Nausea or vomiting during or just after exercise.

- Shortness of breath. You will breathe faster when you exercise, but if you can't seem to get a good breath, you should be concerned.

OTHER LIFESTYLE CHANGES

Smoking

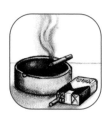

Smoking is a hard habit to break, but it is the single largest risk factor for heart disease. Quitting now is the most important change you can make in your life. Your doctor, cardiac rehabilitation specialist, or even your local phone book can direct you to programs to help you stop smoking. There are many books on the subject and plenty of support groups.

Most people need help to stop smoking, whether emotional support from friends and family or medical support from a doctor. If you need help, talk to your doctor. Do not use nicotine gum, a patch, or any kind of medical aid without discussing it with your doctor first.

Alcohol

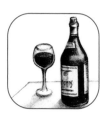

If you are a moderate drinker, you may be able to drink an occasional glass of wine, beer, or mixed drink without problems. In fact, moderate drinking may increase your "good cholesterol" and help your heart. But if you wish to drink, you need to remember:

- Alcohol can cause problems when combined with certain medications, even in small amounts. Ask your pharmacist or doctor about how your medications react with alcohol. Never use an alcoholic drink to wash down a pill.

- Moderate drinking means 1 beer, 4 ounces of wine, or 1 ounce of liquor a day. These amounts may be helpful to your heart, but more than this can cause heart problems—and other problems.

- If you don't drink, don't start.

- If you show any signs of an alcohol problem, talk to a counselor or attend a program that will help you stop drinking.

Stress

There is no way to completely eliminate stress from your life, but it's very important to reduce stress where you can, and to learn to handle it well. When you are stressed, your heart beats faster and your blood pressure goes up.

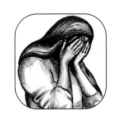

Some things to remember about stress:

- **Learning that you have heart disease is a stressful experience.** Understand that it's normal to feel scared, angry, or sad when you first realize that you have heart disease. Remember, too, that you can make changes in your life—quitting smoking, exercising more, and eating better, for example—that may help you limit your risk and improve your health.

- **Try to avoid situations that are likely to cause anxiety.** For example, if going to the supermarket makes you feel stressed, ask a friend to buy groceries for you, or find a small neighborhood store where there are no crowds.

- **You can't avoid all stressful situations, but you can try not to let them bother you.** Find your own special technique for staying calm in a difficult situation or around people who upset you. For example, many people find "mindful breathing" helpful: Close your eyes and try to concentrate on nothing but inhaling and exhaling slowly.

- **Take care of yourself physically.** Good nutrition, regular exercise, and plenty of sleep can help you stay calm and handle stress more easily.

- **Take care of yourself emotionally.** Talk to your friends and family. Let them know you care about them. Tell them if you are frightened or concerned because of your heart disease. They care for you and want to help you.

- **Relaxing treats may seem like a waste of time or money, but they can mean better health in the long run.** A weekly massage can help you relax and function better. Maybe a funny movie is just what you need. Try turning off the phone and the television for an evening while you listen to soft music and lie quietly, thinking about your favorite place. Even 10 minutes to "de-stress" at the end of the workday can make a big difference in the way you feel.

- **If you need help handling your feelings about heart disease—or other things in your life—see a counselor or therapist.** Sometimes, talking to someone else helps you get a perspective on your own life.

FOLLOW-UP WITH YOUR DOCTOR

Working with your doctor is very important, particularly if you're recovering from surgery or other therapy. Until now you may have seen a doctor only occasionally, for an annual check-up or when you had a touch of the flu. You probably didn't think of you and your doctor as a "team."

But now you are a team—and your team has quite a few other players. In fact, to say "your doctor" is a bit misleading. You may have a number of doctors: your primary care physician (a family practice physician, gynecologist, or internist), a cardiologist, a surgeon (or several of them). Add to that nurses, technicians, anesthesiologists, rehabilitation specialists, pharmacists . . . it may seem like enough for *two* teams.

Communication Triangle

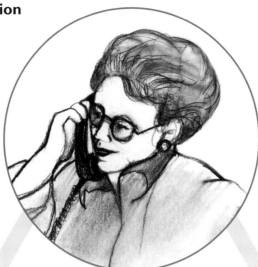

Patient

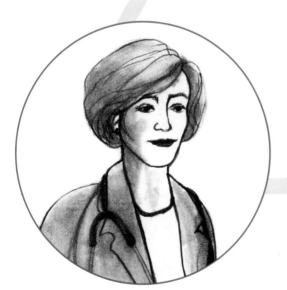

Cardiologist

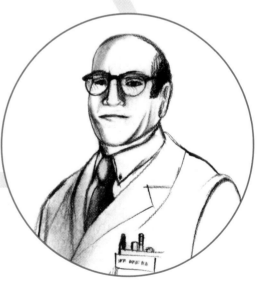

Primary Care Physician

You, your cardiologist, and your primary care physician
should communicate regularly during and after your recovery.

133

So, when you are told to "follow up with your doctor," which doctor are you supposed to talk to? Ask your healthcare team. They will tell you exactly who you should call and when.

It's important that all of your physicians (and their staff members) are communicating. Don't be embarrassed to ask questions about this. It's your heart and your health; be an active "consumer" of medical care.

Your cardiologist and your primary care physician should communicate regularly. Your cardiologist needs to know your medical history, any medical problems you may have, and what medications you are taking. Your primary care physician needs to know what medications the cardiologist has prescribed for your heart disease, what therapy you need, and how your heart disease may affect other parts of your body.

If you have heart surgery, your surgeon will work with your cardiologist to understand your condition before surgery, and the cardiologist will manage your heart care after surgery to see if your condition changes.

You should call your cardiac care physician if:

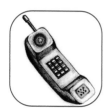

- You have symptoms related to your original heart disease, such as an irregular heart rate, weakness, or chest pain.

- You notice side effects after starting a new heart medication.

- You have been given a prescription for something other than your heart disease.

- You have had surgery, a pacemaker, or another kind of therapy and you notice symptoms that your cardiologist has warned you about.

You should call your primary care physician if:

- You have symptoms that don't seem to be related to your heart disease. You may have the usual viral infections, upset stomachs, and headaches that someone without heart disease gets from time to time.

CHAPTER EIGHT

YOUR HEART IS MORE THAN A BODY PART

If we just look at anatomy, the heart is no more than an organ. A very important organ, one we can't live without, but just a body part, after all. But we don't just look at anatomy. Throughout human history, we have viewed the heart as the center of our emotions. That's something we imagine; it's not literally true. But it often causes us to see heart disease as something beyond a physical disease.

With any serious illness, you must confront the possibility of permanent changes in your life, or even the possibility that you won't live as long as you'd like. Surgery, medication, and lifestyle changes may improve your physical health, but you may need special support to deal with your emotional health.

In this chapter you will learn:

How to cope with your emotions at this time.

How your spiritual beliefs may help you.

If sex is safe after heart disease.

YOUR EMOTIONS

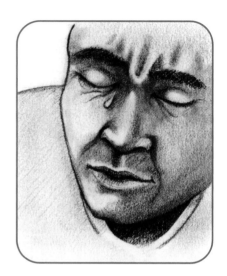

When you learn you have heart disease, you may suddenly have a million things to worry about: Am I going to be okay? How will we pay for my treatment? Can I keep my job? Who's going to mow the lawn if I can't? How do I tell my partner (my parents, my children, my friends)? What are my chances? Will there be side effects from the medication?

A lot of your energy, both physical and emotional, will go toward taking care of yourself and dealing with practical concerns. While all this is going on, you may not pay attention to how you're feeling. Not physically, but emotionally.

Everyone reacts differently on learning that he or she has heart disease. Almost any feeling you have will be "normal." You need to recognize your feelings and accept that it's okay to have them. But you don't want negative feelings to get in the way of your health, or your life.

Fear

Fear may be your first reaction after learning you have heart disease. Am I going to die? Will I have a heart attack if I do anything strenuous? Am I going to get worse?

The first thing to do is get more information. We tend to fear that which we don't understand. Ask your doctor the specifics about your condition. Write your questions down when you think of them, then bring them along to your next appointment. Look for books about your heart disease and discuss what you read with your doctor.

A support group can help. You may feel comforted to meet other people who are worried about the same things you are—and who are learning how to get past their fears.

Talk to your loved ones and let them know what you are afraid of. They can help you get information and keep a healthy perspective.

There may be no way to completely rid yourself of fear. Heart disease is a serious thing, after all. But by addressing your fears head-on, you can learn how to live your life to the fullest, in spite of your heart condition.

Anger

Why me? This is a natural reaction for many people. You eat well, you don't smoke, you exercise. It's not fair that you should get heart disease.

It's okay to indulge your angry feelings for a while—but not if you direct them at other people. It's not your partner's fault, or your parents'. And it's certainly not the fault of the doctor who tells you there's a problem.

If you feel like you need to be angry for a while, try directing it at your disease. "Okay, heart disease, I'm not going to let you get me down. I'm going to do what I can to beat you." This way, you can use your anger as an incentive to make lifestyle changes that will help you control your heart disease.

Anger can get the better of you—and it can make your condition worse. Getting angry often, or staying angry, causes stress. Stress can raise cholesterol, increase heart rate, and create other physical changes that are bad for your heart.

It's best for you to recognize any anger you feel and then do what you must in order to let it go.

Depression

Depression can sneak up on you. You think you're doing okay, handling everything pretty well. But you just don't feel like yourself. You're no longer interested in activities you used to enjoy, or you feel more tired than usual. You withdraw from your friends and loved ones—you just need time by yourself, you think. These changes are sometimes caused by heart disease, medication, or the recovery process following surgery or other treatments. But they may also signify depression.

Depression is not just in your mind, and it is not something you can talk yourself out of. Depression is a combination of emotional and physical changes. If you are depressed, you may need help to handle it.

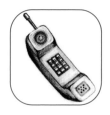

The first step is to recognize that something is wrong. Talk with your doctor about how you're feeling and what physical symptoms you are experiencing. Your doctor can help determine if your heart condition or medication is causing you to feel tired or low. If these factors are ruled out, your doctor can help you figure out the next step. You may be given a referral to a psychiatrist for counseling and antidepressant medication.

People who are depressed often don't recognize it themselves. If loved ones mention that you seem to be acting differently, don't just brush it aside. They are trying to help you. Talk about how you're feeling, and ask what they have noticed. If they describe symptoms of depression, talk to your doctor.

Symptoms of depression can include:

- A sad mood or empty feeling that just won't go away.

- Sleeping too much.

- Sleeping too little, or waking frequently and not being able to get back to sleep.

- Losing interest in the things you used to enjoy.

- Eating too much, or feeling like you don't want to eat at all.

- Gaining or losing weight.

- Irritability or restlessness.

- Fatigue and loss of energy.

- Feeling guilty, hopeless, or worthless.

- Thoughts of suicide or death.

Denial

After learning they have heart disease, some people react by simply not reacting. They refuse to make necessary lifestyle changes and are careless about taking medications or refilling prescriptions. They seem to think that if they ignore their heart disease, it can't hurt them.

Make sure you're not dismissing the seriousness of heart disease. If you have a relatively mild problem now, that's great, but it means that now is the time to do what you can to keep your problem from getting any worse.

If your heart problem is serious, take it seriously. There are people who care about you, and you hurt them as well as yourself if you don't recognize your illness and do what you can to get better.

COMMUNICATION

All of us need to feel connected to others—to a spouse or partner, friends, coworkers, family, a therapist. If you have heart disease, you will struggle to understand an array of confusing emotions, and your need to talk will be very strong.

Communication doesn't always come naturally. You could feel frustrated that the person you're talking to doesn't seem to be listening, or angry because your closest friend feels overwhelmed by your need to talk. To communicate well, there are certain steps you can take:

- **When dealing with medical information, write your questions down ahead of time,** so you won't forget them when you talk to your doctor. Take notes during your doctor appointments, or have someone take notes for you.

- **If you feel like you need to share your deepest thoughts, tell a loved one that you need to talk and ask when would be a good time.** If you are telling your most serious worries to someone who is trying to finish a report on deadline, both of you are likely to feel frustrated.

- **Let your listener know what you need.** If you just want a sympathetic ear, say that you need to vent for a while, but you'd rather not get any advice right now. If you want advice, ask for it. If you want to talk about something completely different from your heart problem, just say so.

- **Be honest, with others and yourself.** You may be embarrassed to tell your doctor that you haven't been following the exercise program, or that you still sneak cigarettes. But not telling the truth can be dangerous, because any information you withhold could affect your treatment plan. With friends and loved ones, you need to be honest about how you feel— even if it will make them worry. "Protecting" others from the truth only builds a wall between you and the ones you love.

- **Practice listening as well as talking.** Remember that the people you love are worried and concerned, too. Maybe they would like to tell you their own fears about your heart disease. Let them know that you're still there for them.

- **Listen to yourself.** Talking to yourself about your heart disease and your emotions is one way to cope. Give yourself a little "you can do it" speech, and pay attention if you seem to be fretting over something in particular. When you listen to yourself—when you acknowledge your most pressing and personal worries—you can begin dealing with the many practical and emotional issues associated with heart disease.

HEALTHY LIFESTYLE

If you feel good physically, you will feel good emotionally, too. To control your heart disease—and to help steer clear of anger, fear, and depression—a healthy diet and regular exercise are essential.

A low-fat, low-sodium, high-fiber diet can give you the energy you need to face the challenges of heart disease. A walk around the block can do a lot toward getting rid of angry feelings. A good night's sleep will refresh you and help you feel more optimistic.

If you are depressed, you may not feel like exercising or watching your diet. But pushing yourself to "live healthy," even when you don't want to, can pay off in the long run. At the very least, when you live a healthy lifestyle, you can feel good that you are taking steps to control your heart disease.

SPIRITUALITY

Many people find it easier to cope with heart disease if they allow themselves to explore their spiritual side. Believing in something beyond yourself can help you put your own life and your own concerns into a broader perspective.

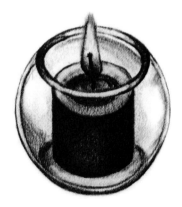

If you belong to an organized religion, attending regular services and participating in your faith community will bring support and fellowship—a great comfort when coping with heart disease. Even if you don't belong to an organized religion, you may find that reading, journaling, meditation, and prayer are important to you now. You may find support by renewing old friendships, or you might simply spend more time thinking about your life and what is important to you.

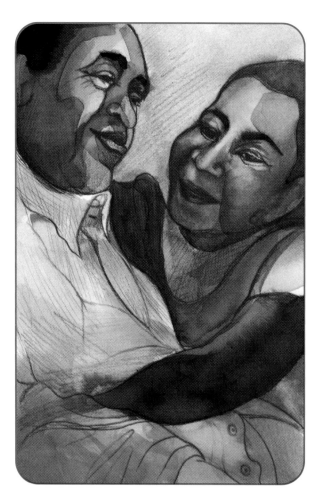

SEXUALITY

If you've just learned that you have heart disease, or if you are recovering from heart surgery, the idea of doing something that will set your heart pounding—like having sex—may be frightening. Or perhaps you're not frightened because, frankly, you just aren't very interested in sex right now. Many people have one or both of those feelings—fear and disinterest—for at least a while.

The phrase "sexual activity" sounds pretty clinical, and most people think it means sexual intercourse. It can be much more, though, including touching, holding, and hugging. You can express love and intimacy in many ways, not all of them leading to intercourse.

There are many myths about sex after heart disease. You've probably heard stories about people who have died "in the midst of passion." Like any other physical activity, sex may cause chest pain, shortness of breath, rapid heart rate, and other symptoms. But the idea that sex can bring on sudden death is simply not true. There is no reason you can't begin sexual activity again when your doctor says it's okay— and when you feel ready.

Is it safe to have sex after heart surgery?

If You Experience Symptoms During Sex

If you have any of the following symptoms during sexual activity, talk to your doctor. A change in medication may correct the problem.

- Chest pain during or after intercourse.

- Shortness of breath for more than 15 minutes after intercourse.

- Racing heartbeat for more than 15 minutes after intercourse.

Loss of Interest

It's perfectly normal to lose interest in sex for a while. You might feel somewhat depressed after being diagnosed with heart disease. Your medications, too, might affect your interest in or ability to have sex. Finally, fears about whether it's safe to have sex—and whether you'll be able to respond the way you used to—can have a profound effect on your sex drive.

Why have I suddenly lost interest in sex?

If you pay attention to your mood swings, you can learn to take advantage of the times you feel good. What causes you to feel blue? What makes you happy? Are you in a better mood before eating or after? Do you have a slump just before you go to bed at night?

Depression is normal. News of heart disease makes you think about your life, your health, the possibility of death. It takes time to come to grips with these. But if you feel depressed for 3 months or more, talk with your doctor about counseling or other therapy.

If you have a sudden change in your ability to have sex, it may be the result of your medication. Ask your doctor if this is a normal side effect and whether adjustments can be made.

One of the best things you can do to make sex a safe part of your life is to get yourself in healthy physical condition. The right kind of aerobic exercise, prescribed by your doctor or therapist, will improve your overall condition and help you feel more confident.

You and your partner may need to adjust your expectations about sex. If you were very active during sexual activity before, you may find that you want something a little calmer now, at least for a while. Or you may need to try new positions that don't put pressure on a surgical incision or a pacemaker.

Many people have trouble adjusting to sex after a heart attack or heart surgery. You and your partner need to talk openly about your feelings and concerns. Nearly everyone worries about being able to perform, hurting the heart, how much is "too much." Even with the best communication, it may take a while before you feel comfortable with sex again. Begin slowly and patiently, gradually increasing your activities at your own pace.

You should not push yourself into sexual activity if you don't feel ready. But if fear or depression are causing you to withdraw from sex altogether, talk to your doctor. He or she may suggest counseling to help you overcome these difficult emotions.

When to Start Having Sex Again

Ask your doctor when it's safe for you to begin having sex. People recovering from a heart attack usually are able to start having sexual intercourse again after 2 or 3 weeks. People who have had heart surgery may start having sex again in 2 to 4 weeks, depending on their condition. Remember, it takes a while to recover from any kind of surgery, and everyone's situation is different. It may take you more time—or less—to feel comfortable with sex again. To put less stress on your heart during sexual intercourse:

- **Choose a time when you feel rested and relaxed,** when you've had time to put aside the usual stresses and worries of the day.

- **Wait at least 2 hours after eating a heavy meal.**

- **If you drink alcohol, always drink in moderation (1 or 2 drinks), and wait 2 to 3 hours after having a drink.**

- **If you take medication for your heart disease, your doctor may recommend taking it before you have sex.** For some people, taking nitroglycerin before having sex can help prevent angina. When your doctor indicates that you are physically ready to start having sexual relations again, be sure to ask about how you should take your medications.

- **Take your time getting there.** Foreplay—kissing, touching, massage—will help you and your heart prepare for the more active part of sexual intercourse.

- **Find a comfortable position that doesn't put pressure on your chest.** You might try lying on your side or back.

CHAPTER NINE

FOR LOVED ONES

If someone you love is coping with heart disease, you may feel selfish thinking about yourself. "I'm fine," you might say. "It's not my disease, after all." True: It's not your disease. Nevertheless, it can dramatically change your life.

This chapter is aimed at partners, children, close friends, parents, and anyone who loves and supports someone with heart disease.

In this chapter you will learn:

What emotions you can expect after your loved one is diagnosed with heart disease.

How to support, not take over, your loved one's recovery.

How to keep yourself healthy.

YOU HAVE FEELINGS, TOO

When a loved one develops heart disease, all of the focus shifts to the patient. There's the fear and uncertainty at the first symptom or diagnosis, the hopefulness—or hopelessness—of treatment, the period of recovery, the lifestyle changes made necessary by the disease.

It makes sense for the focus to be on the patient. He or she needs a lot of emotional support, and maybe a lot of physical support as well. Friends and relatives begin to call or visit your loved one. All of your conversations seem to center on the treatment he or she is getting, the progress he or she has made. Amid the worry and concern, it's easy for you—partner, sibling, parent, child, close friend—to fade into the background.

You try to be supportive and strong, but in doing so, you may end up neglecting yourself in ways that can hurt you—and your loved one—in the long run.

Sometimes you, too, need to have a good cry—or a good laugh. You need to talk about what makes you afraid—and what makes you mad. Sometimes you just need a break.

While it's important to recognize and talk about your own feelings, you may need to protect your loved one. He or she has a lot to deal with, you're right about that. It's hard for a person with heart disease to be as supportive as he or she normally would. If your loved one is a person you confide in, such as your spouse or partner, you may need to look elsewhere for a sympathetic, supportive, and helpful ear.

You may experience a number of emotions while coping with your loved one's heart disease. Some of these emotions are discussed in the pages that follow. You may feel all of them or none of them. Or, you may feel completely different emotions than those described here. Remember, people react very differently during periods of stress.

Fear

You may be afraid that your loved one might die or become permanently disabled. You may fear that you won't have the strength or the courage to go through illness, treatment, and recovery. You may fear that you will be left alone without enough money to keep your home or take care of your children.

You may fear the unknown. What happens next? Will you be caring for an invalid, grieving a death, or getting both of your lives back on track? Sometimes people are great at handling awful circumstances, but they are uncomfortable when they don't know how a situation is going to turn out. With heart disease, nothing is certain. A treatment may hold great promise, but success is never guaranteed.

The saying "We have nothing to fear but fear itself" may seem a bit too simple for the complicated situation that you and your loved one are in. But fear is a crippling emotion. It tends to stop you from taking steps that may improve your situation.

Getting information is one of the best ways to deal with fear. If you are worried about money, now is a good time to look into your savings and expenses and talk with a financial advisor. If you're concerned about your loved one's treatment, ask the doctor questions and do your own research. Taking action won't banish fear altogether, but it can help keep fear under control.

Reassurance from others may help. Talk to friends and family members. They are likely to tell you that everything is going to be fine. It's important for you to hear that, even if you see signs that this will be a very difficult time. You *will* be fine, but you have to deal with some tough issues first.

You need to tell your loved one something about your fears, but you must be careful in doing so. Your loved one has a lot of fear already. It may help your loved one to know that you share some of that fear. But letting your loved one know that you are panicked and need help may only pressure your loved one when he or she is not in a good position to support you.

Resentment

How could you resent someone who is so sick? You may think you are selfish and mean to resent a loved one who is ill with heart disease, but resentment is relatively common.

You may resent your loved one for having ignored advice about diet and exercise, so you blame him or her for allowing this illness to develop. You may resent the time and energy you are expected to spend taking care of your loved one. You may feel exhausted from caregiving and resentful of the amount of attention your loved one receives.

Maybe it's not your loved one you resent, but something else—fate, God, healthy people. *It's not fair!,* you want to shout. *We were good. Why is my loved one ill?*

Resentment is a hard emotion to bury. If you feel it, at some point you are likely to express it. And if you've bottled it up for a while, it can come pouring out in an ugly way.

If you are feeling resentful, you may fear that others will think you are a terrible person. This is a good time to talk to a counselor or someone who has been through a similar situation. Your hospital or clinic may sponsor support groups, or they can refer you to a counselor or therapist who understands what it means to love a person with heart disease. Many employers have employee assistance programs that can direct you to support services and counseling.

Abandonment

Although you might spend all of your time—or what seems like all of your time—with your loved one, you may still feel as if you've been abandoned. He or she is on a "journey" of illness, and you can't really be part of it. Your loved one's full attention is focused on the disease, the treatment, and what it means for the rest of his or her life. Although this person loves you, he or she can't fully be there for you right now—just when you really need his or her support.

If your loved one is your partner or close friend, he or she may be your closest human contact, the one you confide in, the one who has always supported you. And now that's missing.

You are less likely to feel abandoned if you stay involved—or get involved—with other people. Although your loved one may need a lot of your time, you can usually take a few hours here and there to be with other friends or family members, to remind yourself that you are surrounded by people who care about you.

Don't abandon your loved one emotionally because you feel abandoned. Keep up the effort to be close. And don't just talk about the disease. Talk about what's bugging you at work, or how proud you are of the children. Hold hands and hug and use loving words. Sometimes, letting yourself be close can make your relationship even stronger.

Sadness

It's natural to feel sad when someone close to you is ill. You have new emotional and physical demands that are hard to keep up with. One of the most important people in your world isn't feeling well. You may be facing the possible loss of this person.

Your lives are not normal, and you miss that. You want to cry. You want to pull the blankets up over your head and go to sleep.

It's important to understand that you're allowed to be sad sometimes. So let yourself be, within reason. If you need to cry, then go ahead and cry. (Crying can cause physical changes that will make you feel better.) If you want to sleep, sleep late when you can. Reach out to your friends and family—they probably will be very understanding and comforting.

Do try to include some things in your life that make you happy. Go to funny movies (laughter, too, can make you feel better), take walks in pretty places, spend time with friends who are interesting and lively, read bedtime stories to your children—or read to someone else's children.

Depression

Sadness is normal. Depression goes beyond sadness. When you are depressed, you feel a sense of hopelessness. You're not just sad that things are difficult now; you're convinced that things will never be good again.

Some signs of depression are:

How do I know
if I'm depressed?

- Difficulty sleeping. You can't seem to sleep, or you sleep all the time.

- Difficulty eating. You eat too much, or you don't feel like eating at all.

- Weight loss or gain.

- Lack of energy.

- Irritability or restlessness.

- Loss of interest in things you used to enjoy.

- Feelings of worthlessness or hopelessness.

- Thoughts of suicide.

If you think you are suffering from depression, you need to get help. Depression is a real illness that can have serious consequences. Counseling may help, but for some people, medication is the best way to begin dealing with depression.

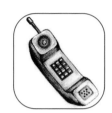

If friends say you don't seem to be yourself, or they wonder aloud whether you are depressed, pay attention. Depressed people see the world as very bleak, and they often do not realize that they are ill.

Guilt

Maybe it was your fault, you think. You could have made her exercise more. You could have cooked healthier meals for him. You didn't want to listen when your loved one said she was under a lot of stress at work. You nudged him to go shovel snow, even though he complained that he didn't feel right.

Guilt is a normal reaction, but you don't want to stay guilty for very long. If you feel guilty, there are two important points you should remember:

- Your loved one made his or her own choices. Yes, maybe you could have made healthier meals, but so could he or she. You put butter on the table, but he or she put it on the bread.

- Some heart disease is no one's fault. Your loved one may have been born with a genetic tendency toward the disease.

Fretting about what you *should* have done is useless. What's important now is what you choose to do next. You cooked unhealthy meals? Well, now you're going to make healthy ones. You didn't encourage your loved one to exercise? You're going to take walks together every day in the future.

HEALTHY WAYS TO DEAL WITH YOUR FEELINGS

Although you need to express your feelings, you don't want to let them get the best of you. The following ideas will help you cope with your emotions:

- **Learn or practice deep breathing exercises.** Sit quietly for a few minutes each day and pay attention to your breathing. Try to clear your mind of thoughts and feelings for this time. Just count your breaths, close your eyes, and be aware of yourself in the moment. This is a basic form of meditation. You may find that it brings you a little peace and lets you get through each day more easily. If it helps, you may want to find a book or audiotape that teaches other meditation techniques.

- **Talk to yourself about how you feel—and recognize that you are okay.** You can say to yourself: "I am really angry with Jim about his getting sick. He never took care of himself, and now I may end up alone because of that." But then you should follow it with something like, "I am angry with Jim, but I know he is even more angry and scared than I am. It's okay for me to be angry right now, but I will get over it so I can help Jim." Or you may say, "I will be very sad if Jim dies; he is the most important person in my life. But I know that I will survive and be able to lead a happy life." This may sound foolish or unrealistic to you, but the point is to avoid "catastrophizing" (telling yourself that things are horrible, that you can't possibly get through it, or that your life will be awful).

- **Talk to other people.** They can give you a reality check and provide support when you need it.

- **Remember what has helped you feel better in the past.** If exercise is your solution to anger, then get to the gym. If pampering yourself is the way you banish sadness, then bring on the bubble bath and the scented candles.

- **Explore your spirituality.** Those with a regular place of worship often find their faith community to be welcoming and supportive. If your spirituality is of a more personal, individual nature, find a quiet place to explore it in your own way.

- **Read helpful books.** The self-help sections in bookstores have grown tremendously over the past decade. A book of meditations or prayers, or a book about others who have struggled with a loved one's illness, can remind you that you are not alone.

SUPPORTING YOUR LOVED ONE

When someone close to you has heart disease, you want to do everything you can to help your loved one cope with the illness, go through treatment, and recover to the fullest extent possible. If your loved one must change his or her diet, you might change yours as well. To encourage your loved one to exercise, you might exercise more yourself.

How can I support my loved one?

There will be medical decisions to make and medical appointments to keep. Try to get as much information as possible in order to understand what is happening to your loved one.

People with heart disease tend to do better if they have someone supporting them and helping them. Having your support can be important to your loved one's recovery and future health.

It's Not Your Responsibility

Some people go way beyond support, however, taking responsibility for their loved one's heart disease as if it were their own. You can help your loved one in many ways, but you can't make him or her do what's best, and you can't make him or her get better.

By preparing low-fat, low-cholesterol meals, you are supporting your loved one. Nagging, criticizing, fretting, or getting angry is not helpful. If your loved one puts butter on his or her bread, or insists on a dish of ice cream for dessert, that's your loved one's choice—and his or her responsibility. If your loved one turns you down every time you suggest going for a walk and getting a little exercise, you will not help by reminding your loved one of how a sedentary life can damage his or her heart.

What if my loved one refuses to change his or her lifestyle?

Some people become so concerned about their loved one that they "overcorrect" in almost every way. They count every calorie, forbid their loved one to do anything even mildly strenuous, and lecture him or her about every choice. Although this is done out of genuine concern, it can do more harm than good. People tend to rebel if they are dictated to. You can actually force your loved one into using unhealthy behaviors as an act of independence.

Controlling heart disease is often a joint effort, but remember, you are not the one running your loved one's life.

Communication

It's easy to get so wrapped up in worrying about your loved one that you forget about good communication. You might end up monitoring the day's progress: Did you take your pills? How are you feeling? What did the doctor say?

Meaningful communication is important now. So is relatively mundane communication. If you have always shared stories about how things went at work, or about the people you saw at the gym, don't stop sharing those stories now. If you've always asked for advice about little things, keep asking. Don't make it seem as if your loved one is no longer an everyday part of your life.

At the same time, you need to talk about the big things, and you need to do it well. Your loved one needs to know what's on your mind. But letting your feelings spill out all over the place may not be the best way to communicate. Remember, communication takes two people, and both need to talk and listen.

Follow these tips for good communication:

- **Pick your time and place.** Don't try to have an important discussion when one of you is tired, or in a hurry to get somewhere, or just having a bad day. And if you have children, don't try to talk over the noise of their activities.

- **Try to use language that doesn't accuse or blame, and stay focused on your own thoughts and feelings.** A comment like, "I get upset when you do things that are not good for your health" is a lot better than, "You make me upset when you do things that are not good for your health." The first simply states how you feel; the second sounds like an accusation.

- **Listen well.** You might try "echoing" or "reflecting," which means repeating what your loved one says to you. This shows your loved one that you are listening and understanding, and it forces you to concentrate on what the other person is saying. If your partner says, "I'm afraid that I will never be able to feel healthy again," you might say back, "You're afraid you won't feel healthy." This can sound artificial at first, but if you and your partner keep practicing, you are likely to improve your ability to communicate.

- **If you think it will help, you and your partner might come up with a plan for talking about important topics.** You can set a specific time and place, and a specific length for the conversation. You can decide to take turns, and you can even set the order in which you talk.

- **Remember to laugh.** Communication is always important, but it doesn't always have to be serious. Sharing humor is an important way to connect with your loved one—and to remind him or her that your lives involve more than coping with heart disease.

STAYING HEALTHY YOURSELF

In taking care of your loved one, it's easy to start neglecting yourself. That's bad for both of you. You need to eat right, get plenty of sleep and exercise, and have a social life with or without your loved one. It's not selfish to take care of yourself. In fact, you might inspire your loved one to do the same.

Diet

That low-fat, low-sodium, high-fiber diet that is so good for someone with heart disease is also good for you. It can help you prevent heart disease in yourself, and it will make you feel better as you go about your life.

We sometimes handle stress by reaching for a candy bar or dishing out a big plate of mashed potatoes loaded with gravy. The words "comfort food" are almost always attached to things that are not very good for us. Instead of a candy bar, grab an orange. Instead of mashed potatoes with gravy, try spaghetti with low-fat tomato sauce. Eat regular meals and keep normal portions.

If you stick to a healthy diet, chances are your loved one will follow. You'll not only keep yourself healthy, you'll help your loved one control his or her heart disease.

Exercise

After taking care of someone else, you may feel like you've had all the exercise you can handle. All you want to do is go to bed. While getting plenty of sleep is important right now, so is regular aerobic exercise.

Walking is the easiest way to get regular exercise. You can walk outdoors in good weather, or inside a shopping mall or fitness club in bad weather. You don't need special clothes or equipment. Just put on a pair of comfortable shoes and put one foot in front of the other.

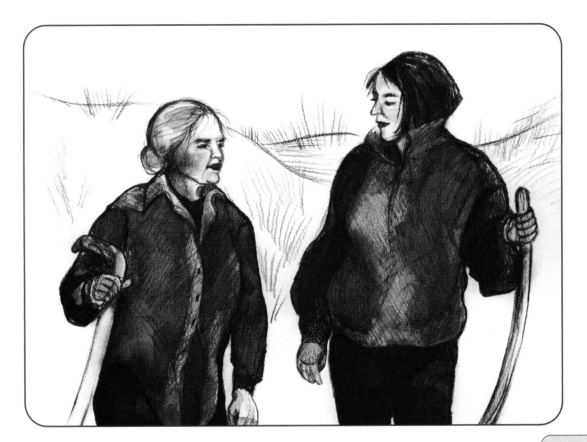

If you walk, your loved one is more likely to walk with you. After one partner has had a heart attack or another symptom of heart disease, many couples have begun taking daily walks together. Besides being good for the person with heart disease, both partners find the walks enjoyable—and both can use that time to remember just how much they like being together.

If you're ready for more than walking, you can join a gym, take up tennis, or learn t'ai chi. Pick exercises that you enjoy; you're more likely to keep on doing them. It's great if your partner can share, but even if he or she can't, you need the exercise. It's important to be fit and strong so you can assist your loved one, if you are able, and protect yourself from injury.

Social Life

Your loved one may be the most important person in your life, but it's not good if he or she is the *only* person in your life. Let friends know that you are interested in socializing. Make sure you see other people at least once a week. No matter how busy you are, you can fit in an hour for coffee with a close friend, or a long walk with your sister.

Tell friends what you want from them. Do you need a shoulder to cry on? Say so. Do you want to talk about something other than your loved one's heart disease? Be clear about that. Your friends will respect your wishes. They want to help, but they may not be sure how.

If your loved one is able, be sure to arrange some social activities with the two of you. Invite friends or family for dinner or a card game. Go to a movie. Remind yourselves that heart disease isn't the only thing in your lives.

SOMETIMES YOU NEED HELP

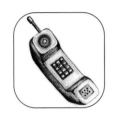

No matter how much you try to support your loved one, you may find the disease more than you can handle. Friends and family are reassuring, but you still feel like you're doing everything wrong. You're tired and scared, and your loved one seems to shut you out at times.

If your clinic or hospital has a support group, take advantage of it. Meeting people who have the same reactions and concerns you do will help you feel that you're not alone—and that you can survive, just as they have.

Your employer may have an employee assistance program that can direct you to counseling. Maybe you just need a "professional" ear to talk to, or maybe you need psychological counseling and medication to cope with anxiety or depression.

Getting help is not a weakness. In fact, it takes quite a bit of strength to admit that you can't cope with your loved one's disease without some help.

ADDITIONAL RESOURCES

BOOKS

Alcohol and Tobacco

American Cancer Society. *American Cancer Society's "Fresh Start": 21 Days to Stop Smoking.* New York: Simon and Schuster, 1986.

American Lung Association, Edwin B. Fisher, and C. Everett Koop. *Lung Association 7 Steps to a Smoke-Free Life.* New York: John Wiley and Sons, 1998.

Gebhardt, Jack. *Help Your Smoker Quit: A Radically Happy Strategy for Nonsmoking Parents, Kids, Spouses, and Friends.* Minneapolis: Fairview Press, 1998.

Holmes, Peter, and Peggy Holmes. *Out of the Ashes: Help for People Who Have Stopped Smoking.* Minneapolis: Fairview Press, 1992.

Mumey, Jack. *The New Joy of Being Sober: A Book for Recovering Alcoholics and Those Who Love Them.* Minneapolis: Fairview Press, 1994.

Cookbooks

American Heart Association. *American Heart Association Low-Salt Cookbook: A Complete Guide to Reducing Sodium and Fat in the Diet.* New York: Times Books, 1995.

American Heart Association. *American Heart Association Low-Fat, Low-Cholesterol Cookbook: Heart-Healthy, Easy-to-Make Recipes That Taste Great.* New York: Times Books, 1998.

American Heart Association. American Heart Association Quick and Easy Cookbook: More Than 200 Healthful Recipes You Can Make in Minutes. New York: Times Books, 1998.

Crocker, Betty. *Betty Crocker's Best of Healthy and Hearty Cooking: More Than 400 Recipes Your Family Will Love.* Foster City, Calif.: IDG Books Worldwide, 1998.

Crocker, Betty. *Betty Crocker's New Choices Cookbook: More Than 500 Great-Tasting, Easy Recipes for Eating Right.* Foster City, Calif.: IDG Books Worldwide, 1993.

Havala, Suzanne. *Being Vegetarian (The American Dietetic Association Nutrition Now Series)*. New York: John Wiley and Sons, 1998.

Melina, Vesanto, Brenda Davis, and Victoria Harrison. *Becoming Vegetarian: The Complete Guide to Adopting a Healthy Vegetarian Diet*. Summertown, Tenn.: Book Publishing Company, 1995.

Piscatella, Joseph P. *Don't Eat Your Heart Out*. New York: Workman, 1994.

Ponichtera, Brenda J., and Janice Staver (illustrator). *Quick and Healthy Recipes and Ideas*. The Dalles, Oreg.: Scaledown, 1991.

Show, Diana. *Almost Vegetarian: A Primer for Cooks Who Are Eating Vegetarian Most of the Time, Chicken and Fish Some of the Time, and Altogether Well All of the Time*. New York: Crown, 1994.

Spitler, Sue, and Linda Yoakam. *1001 Low-Fat Vegetarian Recipes*. Chicago: Surrey Books, 1997.

Wasserman, Debra, and Reed Mangels. *Simply Vegan: Quick Vegetarian Meals*. Baltimore: Vegetarian Resource Group, 1999.

Fitness and Nutrition

American Dietetic Association. *Cut The Fat: More Than 500 Easy and Enjoyable Ways to Reduce the Fat from Every Meal*. New York: HarperCollins, 1996.

American Heart Association. *American Heart Association Fitting in Fitness: Hundreds of Simple Ways to Put More Physical Activity into Your Life*. New York: Times Books, 1997.

American Heart Association. *The Healthy Heart Walking Book: The American Heart Association Walking Program*. Foster City, Calif.: IDG Books Worldwide, 1995.

Anderson, Jean, and Barbara Deskins. *The Nutrition Bible: The Comprehensive, No-Nonsense Guide to Foods, Nutrients, Additives, Preservatives, Pollutants, and Everything Else We Eat and Drink*. New York: William Morrow and Company, 1997.

Bland, John H., with Jenna Colby. *The Complete Mall Walker's Handbook: Walking for Fun and Fitness*. Minneapolis: Fairview Press, 1999.

Diabetes Education and Self-Management Program, Fairview-University Medical Center. "Guide to Carbohydrate Counting." Minneapolis: Fairview Publications, 1999.

Duyff, Roberta Larson. *The American Dietetic Association's Complete Food and Nutrition Guide*. New York: John Wiley and Sons, 1998.

Franz, Marion. *Fast Food Facts: The Original Guide for Fitting Fast Food into a Healthy Lifestyle*. Minneapolis: IDC Publishing, 1997.

Gershoff, Stanley N., and Catherine Whitney. *The Tufts University Guide to Total Nutrition*. New York: HarperCollins, 1996.

Herbert, Victor, and Genell Subak-Sharpe, editors. *Total Nutrition: The Only Guide You'll Ever Need*. New York: St. Martin's Press, 1995.

Margen, Sheldon, and Steve Mays (photographer). *The Wellness Encyclopedia of Food and Nutrition: How to Buy, Store and Prepare Every Variety of Fresh Food*. New York: Rebus, 1999.

Netzer, Corinne T. *The Complete Book of Food Counts*. New York: Dell Publishing, 1997.

Pennington, Jean A. T., Anne De Planter Bowes, and Helen N. Church. *Bowes and Church's Food Values of Portions Commonly Used*. Philadelphia: Lippincott Williams and Wilkins, 1997.

Tribole, Evelyn. *Eating on the Run*. Champaign, Ill.: Human Kinetics, 1991.

Medical Information

American Heart Association. *American Heart Association Guide to Heart Attack Treatment, Recovery, and Prevention*. New York: Times Books, 1998.

American Heart Association. *American Heart Association's Your Heart: An Owner's Manual*. New York: Prentice Hall, 1995.

Dyken, Mark L., and J. Donald Easton. *American Heart Association Family Guide to Stroke Treatment, Recovery, and Prevention*. New York: Times Books, 1996.

McGoon, Michael D. *Mayo Clinic Heart Book*. New York: William Morrow and Company, 1993.

Medical Economics Company. *The PDR Family Guide to Prescription Drugs*. New York: Three Rivers Press, 1999.

Rybacki, James J., and James W. Long. *The Essential Guide to Prescription Drugs 2000*. New York: Harper Resource, 1999.

Sullivan, Donald. *The American Pharmaceutical Association's Guide to Prescription Drugs.* New York: Signet, 1998.

United States Pharmacopeia. *The Complete Drug Reference: 2000 Edition.* Yonkers, N.Y.: Consumer Reports Books, 1999.

NEWSLETTERS/MAGAZINES

Consumer Reports on Health
Customer Service
P.O. Box 52148
Boulder, Colorado 80321
(800) 333-9784
https://www.neodata.com/ConsumerReports/crohusa.html

Cooking Light Magazine
P.O. Box 830549
Birmingham, Alabama 35282-9558
(800) 336-0125
http://www.cookinglight.com

Diabetes Forecast
American Diabetes Association
1701 North Beauregard Street
Alexandria, Virginia 22311
(800) 806-7801
http://www.diabetes.org

Environmental Nutrition Newsletter
P.O. Box 420235
Palm Coast, Florida 32142-0235
(800) 829-5384

Mayo Clinic Health Letter
Subscription Services
P.O. Box 53887
Boulder, Colorado 80321
(800) 333-9038
http://www.mayo.edu/pub-rst/healthlt.html

Nutrition Action Healthletter
Center for Science in the Public Interest
1875 Connecticut Avenue N.W.
Suite 300
Washington, D.C. 20009
(202) 332-9110
http://www.cspinet.org

Tufts University *Health and Nutrition Letter*
P.O. Box 420235
Palm Coast, Florida 32142-0235
(800) 274-7581
http://www.healthletter.tufts.edu./

University of California at Berkeley *Wellness Letter*
P.O. Box 420148
Palm Coast, Florida 32142
(800) 829-9080

ORGANIZATIONS

Alcohol, Drugs, and Tobacco

American Lung Association
1740 Broadway
New York, New York 10019
(212) 315-8700
(800) LUNG-USA
http://www.lungusa.org

National Clearinghouse for Alcohol and Drug Information
P.O. Box 2345
Rockville, Maryland 20847-2345
(800) 729-6686
http://www.health.org

National Council on Alcoholism and Drug Dependence
12 West 21st Street
Seventh Floor
New York, New York 10010
(212) 206-6670
(800) 622-2255
http://www.ncadd.org

Cardiac Rehabilitation

American Academy of Physical Medicine and Rehabilitation
One IBM Plaza
Suite 2500
Chicago, Illinois 60611-3604
(312) 464-9700
http://www.aapmr.org

National Rehabilitation Information Center
100 Wayne Avenue
Suite 800
Silver Spring, Maryland 20910
(301) 562-2400
(800) 346-2742
http://www.naric.com

Diabetes

African American Program
American Diabetes Association
Customer Service
1701 North Beauregard Street
Alexandria, Virginia 22311
(800) DIA-BETES
http://www.diabetes.org/africanamerican

American Diabetes Association
1701 North Beauregard Street
Alexandria, Virginia 22311
(800) DIA-BETES
http://www.diabetes.org

National Diabetes Information Clearinghouse
One Information Way
Bethesda, Maryland 20892-3560
(301) 654-3327
http://www.niddk.nih.gov/health/diabetes/ndic.htm

Fitness and Nutrition
American Dietetic Association
216 West Jackson Boulevard
Chicago, Illinois 60606-6995
(800) 877-1600
(800) 366-1655 (Consumer Nutrition Hotline)

Weight-Control Information Network
1 WIN Way
Bethesda, Maryland 20892-3665
(301) 984-7378
(800) WIN-8098
http://www.niddk.nih.gov/NutritionDocs.html

Heart Condition
American Heart Association
7272 Greenville Avenue
Dallas, Texas 75231
(800) AHA-USA1 (Heart and Stroke)
(888) MY-HEART (Women's Heart Health)
http://www.americanheart.org

National Heart, Lung, and Blood Institute
P.O. Box 30105
Bethesda, Maryland 20824-0105
(301) 592-8573
http://www.nhlbi.nih.gov

Mental Health

American Psychiatric Association
1400 K. Street N.W.
Washington, D.C. 20005
(202) 682-6000
http://www.psych.org

American Psychological Association
750 First Street, N.E.
Washington, D.C. 20002-4242
(202) 336-5500
(800) 374-2721
http://www.apa.org

National Mental Health Association
1021 Prince Street
Alexandria, Virginia 22314-2971
(703) 684-7722
(800) 969-6642
http://www.nmha.org

Stroke

American Stroke Association
A Division of American Heart Association
7272 Greenville Avenue
Dallas, Texas 75231
(800) UHA-USA1
http://www.americanheart.org

National Institute of Neurological Disorders and Stroke (NINDS)
Information Office
Building 31, Room 8A-O6
31 Center Drive MSC 2540
Bethesda, Maryland 20892-2540
(301) 496-5751
(800) 352-9424
http://www.ninds.nih.gov

National Stroke Association
9707 E. Easter Lane
Englewood, Colorado 80112-3747
(303) 649-1328
(800) STR-OKES
http://www.stroke.org

Support Groups
Mended Hearts
7272 Greenville Avenue
Dallas, Texas 75231-4596
(800) AHA-USA1
http://www.mendedhearts.org

INDEX